W0106463

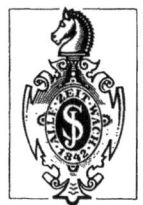

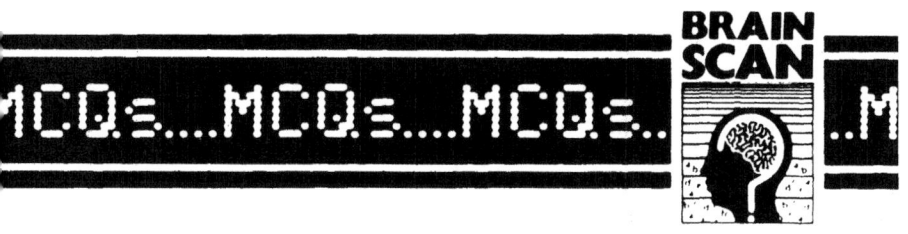

Kevin P. Gibbin · Patrick J. Bradley

Ear, Nose and Throat Disease

Springer-Verlag
London Berlin Heidelberg New York
Paris Tokyo Hong Kong

Kevin P. Gibbin, FRCS
Consultant Otolaryngologist, Department of
Otolaryngology, University Hospital, Queen's
Medical Centre, Nottingham NG7 2UH, UK

Patrick J. Bradley, FRCS
Consultant Otolaryngologist and Head and Neck Oncologist,
Department of Otolaryngology, University Hospital,
Queen's Medical Centre, Nottingham NG7 2UH, UK

Publisher's note: The "Brainscan" logo is reproduced by courtesy of The
Editor, *Geriatric Medicine*, Modern Medicine GB Ltd.

ISBN 978-3-540-19559-7   ISBN 978-1-4471-1699-8 (eBook)
DOI 10.1007/978-1-4471-1699-8

British Library Cataloguing in Publication Data
Gibbin, Kevin P. *1945–*
Ear, nose and throat disease.   1. Man. Ears, nose and throat. Diseases
I. Title   II. Bradley, Patrick, *1949–*   III. Series   617'.51
ISBN 978-3-540-19559-7 *W. Germany*

Library of Congress Cataloging-in-Publication Data
Gibbin, Kevin P., 1945–
Ear, nose, and throat disease/Kevin P. Gibbin, Patrick Bradley.
p.   cm. — (Brainscan MCQ's)
ISBN 978-3-540-19559-7
1. Otolaryngology—Examinations, questions, etc.   I. Bradley, Patrick,
1949–   .   II. Title.   III. Series.   [DNLM: 1. Otorhinolaryngologic
Diseases—examination questions.   WV 18 G438e] RF57.G53   1989
617.5'1'0076—dc20   DNLM/DLC   for Library of Congress   89-11312
                                                                    CIP

© Springer-Verlag Berlin Heidelberg 1989

Filmset by Macmillan India Ltd., Bangalore 25

2128/3830-543210 (Printed on acid-free paper)

Preface

This book was conceived as a means of learning by inquiring—self testing carried out conscientiously is an effective way of acquiring knowledge. A wrongly answered question should stimulate the examinee to return to his books to discover the correct answer, although it should be noted that in a number of cases we have annotated brief comments.

We hope the book will be of benefit to a number of learners in otolaryngology: medical students, house officers and nurses undergoing post-basic training. We hope also that it may help general-practitioner trainees, for whom otolaryngology presents a significant workload.

We recognise that this book must be complementary to standard textbooks but our aspirations remain that the student will gain even greater benefit from his efforts by spending some time in self assessment.

Nottingham   Kevin P. Gibbin
1989   Patrick J. Bradley

Contents

1. Ear

Q.1.1 **In a normal ear**

    a. the membrana tensa and membrana flaccida both contain three distinct layers: epithelial, fibrous and mucosal

    b. the long process of the incus can never be seen through an intact drum

    c. the tip of the long process of the incus articulates with the head of the stapes via a synarthrosis

    d. the incudomallear joint is a synovial joint

    e. in a neonate or very young baby, in order to visualise the tympanic membrane the pinna needs to be gently retracted superiorly to straighten and widen the external auditory canal

Q.1.2 **In a normal ear**

    a. tensor tympani and stapedius muscles are innervated by the motor branch of the maxillary nerve

    b. the role of stapedius is to alter the movement of stapes in response to loud sounds

    c. levels of discomfort and sound intolerance may be reached at 115–120 dB

    d. loss of the pinna or abnormalities of the external auditory canal may result in reduced hearing

    e. the action of stapedius may be detected by tympanometry

Q.1.3 **Regarding the anatomy of the ear:**

    a. The geniculate ganglion is part of the autonomic nervous system containing ganglion cells of nerves supplying the lacrimal gland

    b. Jacobson's nerve is a branch of the trigeminal

    c. The external auditory canal receives sensory innervation from the cranial nerves V, VII, X

    d. The eustachian tube is actively opened by tensor palati and levator palati muscles

    e. The promontory of the middle ear is a bulge caused by the lateral semicircular canal

For answers see over

Answers

A.1.1 a. F—The membrana tensa consists of three distinct layers, as noted; the membrana flaccida lacks the fibrous middle layer.

        b. F—The outline of the long process of the incus can frequently be seen through a completely normal drum; if an ear drum is retracted the long process may be very clearly outlined by the retraction.

        c. F—The incudostapedial joint is a synovial joint.

        d. T

        e. F—In neonates and very young children the pinna needs to be retracted inferiorly in order to straighten and widen the ear canal.

A.1.2 a. F—Tensor tympani is innervated by a branch from the mandibular nerve. Stapedius is innervated by the facial nerve.

        b. T

        c. T

        d. T

        e. T

A.1.3 a. T

        b. F—Jacobson's nerve is the aural branch of the IXth nerve.

        c. T

        d. T

        e. F—The promontory of the middle ear is caused by the basal turn of the cochlea.

Q.1.4 In the inner ear

a. the semicircular canals provide the vestibular statoreceptors
b. the neuroepithelium of the labyrinth connects with the nuclei of the external ocular muscles via the inferior colliculus
c. the cochlear nerve runs through the internal auditory meatus and the cerebellopontine angle to the pons
d. the saccule and utricle detect movement in the vertical and horizontal planes respectively
e. perilymph and endolymph are identical extracellular fluids

Q.1.5 The facial nerve runs through

a. the fallopian canal
b. the parotid gland
c. the middle ear
d. the submandibular gland
e. between the bellies of digastricus

Q.1.6 In facial palsy due to upper motor lesions, unlike that resulting from lower motor lesions,

a. muscle atrophy is present
b. emotional facial movement remains intact
c. forehead movement is paralysed on the same side as the lesion
d. history is helpful in diagnosis
e. there are associated symptoms

Q.1.7 When syringing an ear

a. dizziness developing within 10 seconds may be ignored
b. inquiry should always be made in order to establish whether the ear is known to be perforated
c. the water should preferably be 7 °C *below* body temperature
d. the water should preferably be 7 °C *above* body temperature
e. discharge is *always* a contraindication

For answers see over

Answers

A.1.4 a. F—The semicircular canals detect motion.

b. F—The inferior colliculus is a nucleus in the auditory tract. It is a centre for auditory and possibly some vestibular reflexes. The vestibular apparatus is connected with the nerves to the external ocular muscles via the medial longitudinal bundle.

c. T

d. F—The saccule and utricle are statoreceptors and detect position in space.

e. F—Both are extracellular fluids, but perilymph tends to be rich in sodium and low in potassium, whereas endolymph tends to be rich in potassium and low in sodium.

A.1.5 a. T

b. T

c. T—The fallopian canal is the horizontal portion of the course of the facial nerve through the middle ear.

d. F

e. F

A.1.6 a. F—Muscle atrophy occurs only with lower motor lesions.

b. T

c. F—Movement is intact in upper motor lesions.

d. T

e. T

A.1.7 a. F—Dizziness should never be ignored when syringing an ear. However, the most likely cause is a caloric effect of using water that is either too hot or too cold.

b. T

c. F—The water should be *at* body temperature.

d. F

e. F—Occasionally syringing may be used in cases of otitis externa as long as the integrity of the drum can be established.

Q.1.8 **Referred pain in one ear may be via**

a. the hypoglossal nerve
b. the auriculotemporal nerve
c. Jacobson's nerve
d. the greater auricular nerve
e. the abducent nerve

Q.1.9 **Unilateral earache in the absence of otitis may be from**

a. temporomandibular joint dysfunction
b. carcinoma of piriform fossa
c. adenoid enlargement
d. allergic rhinitis
e. quinsy

Q.1.10 **The differential diagnosis of a swelling in the ear canal should include**

a. mumps
b. aural polyp
c. sebaceous cyst
d. osteoma
e. carcinoma

Q.1.11 **A very tender nodule on the helix of the pinna may be due to**

a. carcinoma, either basal cell or squamous
b. sebaceous cyst
c. chondrodermatitis nodularis helicis
d. chondroma
e. aberrant parotid tissue

Q.1.12 **Keratosis obturans**

a. is a premalignant condition
b. is always associated with underlying cholesteatoma
c. is an accumulation of squamous debris in the ear canal causing blockage of the canal
d. is part of Kartagener's triad
e. needs emergency mastoid surgery

For answers see over

Answers

A.1.8 a. F
         b. T
         c. T
         d. T
         e. F

A.1.9 a. T
         b. T
         c. F
         d. F
         e. T

A.1.10 a. F
         b. T
         c. T
         d. T
         e. T

A.1.11 a. T
         b. F—Sebaceous cysts are rarely tender.
         c. T
         d. F—These are usually painless.
         e. F

A.1.12 a. F
         b. F
         c. T
         d. F—Kartagener's triad is sinusitis, bronchiectasis and dextrocardia.
         e. F

Q.1.13   The following are contraindications to syringing an ear:

a. Chronic suppurative otitis media
b. Otitis externa
c. Ménière's disorder
d. Total meatal atresia
e. Keratosis obturans

Q.1.14   Otitis externa may cause

a. earache
b. keratosis obturans
c. meningitis
d. trismus
e. perichondritis of the pinna

Q.1.15   Otitis externa may be

a. localised
b. diffuse
c. associated with diabetes and proceed to meningitis, brain abscess and death
d. due to chronic sinusitis
e. treated by cautery with silver nitrate

Q.1.16   The treatment of otitis externa should always be by

a. syringing
b. suction toilet
c. gentian-violet applied topically
d. topical antibiotics
e. intramuscular penicillin injections

Q.1.17   Acute furunculosis of the ear canal should be treated by

a. intramuscular antibiotics
b. topical antibiotics
c. glycerine and ichthammol wicks and local heat
d. analgesia as required
e. incision and drainage using a pointed stick

For answers see over

Answers

A.1.13   a.   T
           b.   F
           c.   F
           d.   T
           e.   T—Keratosis obturans is a condition in which there is extensive build-up of epithelial debris in the ear canal, and syringing may be impossible and is contraindicated because of the uncertainty as to whether there is underlying otitis media.

A.1.14   a.   T
           b.   F—Keratosis is a form of otitis externa.
           c.   F
           d.   T
           e.   T

A.1.15   a.   T
           b.   T
           c.   T—This is called malignant or necrotising otitis externa.
           d.   F
           e.   F

A.1.16   a.   F—However, syringing may sometimes be of benefit in an ear with otitis externa, as long as there is no underlying middle ear pathology.
           b.   T
           c.   F—However, gentian-violet has in the past been used for topical treatment of otitis externa.
           d.   T—But the mainstay of treatment is by appropriate toilet to the ear.
           e.   F—But systemic antibiotics may *sometimes* be necessary.

A.1.17   a.   F
           b.   F
           c.   T
           d.   T
           e.   F

Q.1.18 **Severe earache with a postaural swelling, malaise and pyrexia may be due to**

  a. a furuncle in the ear canal
  b. otosclerosis
  c. acute mastoiditis
  d. cholesteatoma
  e. Ramsay Hunt syndrome

Q.1.19 **In suspected acute mastoiditis the treatment required may include**

  a. radical mastoidectomy
  b. cortical mastoidectomy
  c. intravenous antibiotics
  d. antibiotic ear drops
  e. antihistamines

Q.1.20 **In cases of suspected acute mastoiditis**

  a. the diagnosis is usually easily made
  b. mastoid X-rays are often necessary to help establish the diagnosis
  c. the disorder is easily differentiated from other ear conditions such as a boil in the ear canal
  d. there is always a clear history of a preceding upper respiratory tract infection
  e. antibiotics should not be administered until a bacteriology swab report is available

Q.1.21 **The following statements apply to the assessment of the hearing of infants and young children**

  a. Distraction testing is usually possible by age 6 months
  b. Details of developmental milestones are important
  c. Questioning the parents is unnecessary
  d. Brainstem electrical responses should be tested routinely in all children over age 1 year
  e. Sound-treated rooms are essential

For answers see over

Answers

A.1.18 a. T
b. F
c. T—Furunculosis in the external auditory canal is occasionally difficult to differentiate from acute mastoiditis, the diagnosis sometimes resting on radiological evidence.
d. F
e. F—Ramsay Hunt syndrome is herpes zoster oticus and typically presents with earache, vesication in the canal, deafness and a facial palsy.

A.1.19 a. F
b. T
c. T
d. F
e. F

A.1.20 a. F—The diagnosis may sometimes be very difficult to establish and the disorder difficult to differentiate from, for example, acute furunculosis.
b. T
c. F
d. F
e. F

A.1.21 a. T—The health visitor hearing screening test is typically carried out between ages 6 and 9 months
b. T
c. F—Medical history from the parents is essential in assessing the hearing of any young child.
d. F
e. T—It is essential to avoid distracting outside sounds while carrying out distraction testing in children.

Q.1.22   The Rinne test

a. localises to the good ear in unilateral sensorineural deafness
b. will usually distinguish between a 40 dB conductive and a 40 dB sensorineural deafness
c. will be negative in all cases of conductive deafness
d. will demonstrate a false negative result in mild and moderate unilateral sensorineural deafness but not in severe or profound cases
e. should always be masked by using a Barany box

Q.1.23   Tuning fork tests

a. should be carried out routinely before any middle ear surgery
b. are carried out using the 256 Hz tuning fork
c. can be used to diagnose a "dead" ear
d. can only be carried out in a sound-treated room
e. may help to diagnose noise induced hearing loss

Q.1.24   In audiology

a. glue ear is associated with normal air conduction thresholds
b. presbyacusis is usually associated with a high tone sensorineural loss
c. acoustic neuroma is associated with normal bone conduction but decreased air conduction
d. with a dead ear, the audiogram may show a "shadow" curve
e. Ménière's syndrome is classically associated with a high tone perceptive deafness.

Q.1.25   Pure tone audiometry

a. must always be carried out in a soundproof room
b. is a reliable indicator of hearing disability and handicap
c. may be carried out in children from approximately 3 years of age
d. demonstrates a conductive hearing loss if bone conduction is better than air conduction
e. is a test of hearing threshold for discrete pure tones

For answers see over

Answers

A.1.22 a. T
  b. T
  c. F—A minimum of 20 to 25 dB air-bone gap is essential for conversion of the Rinne test from positive to negative.
  d. F—A false negative result is present in severe or profound unilateral hearing loss, the Rinne test being negative in the affected ear because of cross-skull transmission to the good cochlea.
  e. F—But masking may be necessary in the case of a unilateral hearing loss.

A.1.23 a. T
  b. F—Usually the 512 Hz tuning fork is used; the 256 and 128 Hz tuning forks may cause vibrotactile stimulation.
  c. F—Diagnosis rests on audiometry, but tuning fork testing may give a strong indication.
  d. F
  e. F

A.1.24 a. T—Glue ear may be associated with normal air conduction audiometry.
  b. T
  c. F—Acoustic neuroma commonly presents with a unilateral sensorineural hearing loss; audiometry will therefore show decrease in both bone conduction and air conduction.
  d. T
  e. F—In Ménière's syndrome the hearing loss is typically low tone or flat in its early phases.

A.1.25 a. F—Ideally it should be carried out in a sound treated or soundproofed room, but in certain circumstances a quiet room is acceptable.
  b. F—Pure tone audiometry indicates only the threshold of hearing for pure tones and does not measure more complex functions of hearing.
  c. T
  d. T
  e. T

Q.1.26 A normal tympanogram will show

a. a pressure compliance peak at ± 50 mm water
b. a pressure compliance peak at ± 50 mm mercury
c. a flat trace
d. a peak at - 150 mm mercury
e. a steadily rising curve with increasing pressure

Q.1.27 Tympanometry may help diagnose

a. secretory otitis
b. the site of the lesion in cases of facial palsy
c. presbyacusis
d. eustachian tube dysfunction
e. Goldenhar's syndrome

Q.1.28 The following may predispose to secretory otitis media:

a. Down's syndrome
b. Cleft palate
c. Endolymphatic hydrops
d. Carcinoma of the nasopharynx
e. Coryza

Q.1.29 Tympanometry in secretory otitis media will show

a. a pressure compliance peak at − 100 mm mercury
b. a flat trace
c. a pressure compliance peak of about 2 ml at ± 50 mm water
d. no tracing because compliance is zero
e. a steeply peaked tracing at − 400 mm mercury

Q.1.30 Secretory otitis may cause

a. normal hearing
b. a hearing loss averaging about 30 dB.
c. tympanosclerosis
d. educational difficulties
e. deafness in children under 1 year old

For answers see over

Answers

A.1.26 a. T
   b. F
   c. F—A flat trace is indicative of middle ear effusion.
   d. F
   e. F

A.1.27 a. T
   b. T—If stapedius is affected.
   c. F
   d. T
   e. F

A.1.28 a. T
   b. T
   c. F
   d. T—Unilateral secretory otitis in adults should always arouse a suspicion of nasopharyngeal carcinoma.
   e. T

A.1.29 a. F
   b. T
   c. F—This is a normal result.
   d. F
   e. F

A.1.30 a. T
   b. T
   c. T
   d. T
   e. T—Secretory otitis is the commonest cause of deafness in children, including those under age 1 year.

Q.1.31 Deafness in children under 2 years old is most commonly caused by

a. cholesteatoma
b. glue ear
c. otosclerosis
d. wax in the external meatus
e. neonatal jaundice

Q.1.32 Grommets

a. are inserted to drain fluid from the middle ear
b. allow the middle ear to be ventilated normally
c. may be useful in Ménière's disorder
d. may cause changes in the tympanic membrane
e. must be removed after 6 months

Q.1.33 Secretory otitis media (glue ear) commonly causes

a. sensorineural deafness
b. otorrhoea
c. conductive deafness
d. otalgia
e. vertigo

Q.1.34 In secretory otitis

a. antibiotics may sometimes effect a cure
b. antibiotics should never be used
c. mucolytics will always help the hearing
d. tinnitus may be a symptom
e. there may be severe earache

Q.1.35 Treatment for secretory otitis in childhood should include

a. myringoplasty
b. adenoidectomy
c. tonsillectomy
d. myringotomy, with or without insertion of a grommet
e. provision of a hearing aid

For answers see over

Answers

A.1.31 a. F
           b. T
           c. F
           d. F
           e. F

A.1.32 a. F—Grommets are ventilating tubes.
           b. T
           c. T—The mechanism is uncertain and there may be a large psychogenic effect.
           d. T—Changes in the tympanic membrane are not at all uncommon after insertion of grommets.
           e. F—Grommets do not routinely need to be removed unless persistent infection is present.

A.1.33 a. F
           b. F
           c. T
           d. T
           e. T—Unsteadiness in young children may be found in association with secretory otitis media.

A.1.34 a. T—Reports have suggested that the use of Septrin may be beneficial.
           b. F
           c. F—Mucolytics probably have no beneficial effect.
           d. T
           e. F—Earache is a common feature of secretory otitis but is rarely severe.

A.1.35 a. F—Myringoplasty is an operation to close a perforated eardrum.
           b. T—Adenoidectomy probably assists in the management of secretory otitis.
           c. F
           d. T
           e. T

Q.1.36 Complications of secretory otitis media may include

a. otosclerosis
b. tympanosclerosis
c. cholesteatoma
d. retraction pockets in the tympanic membrane
e. meningitis

Q.1.37 In secretory otitis media the fluid in the middle ear may be

a. thick and mucoid
b. thin and serous
c. bloodstained
d. thick and turbid
e. dark blue

Q.1.38 The tympanic membrane in secretory otitis may be

a. retracted
b. almost normal in appearance
c. perforated
d. blue
e. atrophic, with an atelectatic middle ear

Q.1.39 In secretory otitis

a. the child may complain of earache
b. the child may be prone to recurrent acute suppurative otitis media
c. pain is not a presenting symptom
d. the child may present with a persistent discharge from both ears
e. a history of maternal rubella may be elicited

Q.1.40 In a child of 6 years with secretory otitis

a. hearing may be normal
b. the teachers will always notice a hearing loss
c. meningitis may develop
d. surgical treatment is usually required
e. socioeconomic group may help to determine management

For answers see over

Answers

A.1.36 a. F—Otosclerosis is a disorder of the otic capsule involving growth of new bone, which causes fixation of the stapes footplate.
       b. T
       c. T
       d. T
       e. F

A.1.37 a. T
       b. T
       c. T
       d. T
       e. F

A.1.38 a. T
       b. T
       c. F
       d. T
       e. T

A.1.39 a. T
       b. T
       c. F
       d. F
       e. F

A.1.40 a. T
       b. F—A child with secretory otitis may have a hearing loss but this may not be picked up by the teacher even though the child's performance may be substandard.
       c. F
       d. F—Surgical treatment is required in only a very small percentage of children with secretory otitis.
       e. T—Children with secretory otitis from lower socioeconomic groups may need to be managed more actively.

Q.1.41 **Acute suppurative otitis media in a child of 18 months**

a. may be predisposed to by chronic secretory otitis media
b. always causes a tympanic perforation
c. causes cholesteatoma
d. should be treated by myringotomy and insertion of a grommet
e. may present with diarrhoea and vomiting

Q.1.42 **The following organisms commonly cause acute suppurative otitis media:**

a. *Pneumococcus*
b. *Staphylococcus albus*
c. *Haemophilus influenzae*
d. *Pseudomonas pyogenes*
e. *Neisseria meningitidis*

Q.1.43 **The following may develop as a complication of acute suppurative otitis media:**

a. Chronic suppurative otitis media
b. Chronic secretory otitis media
c. Persistent perforation of the membrana tensa
d. Persistent attic perforation
e. Facial palsy

Q.1.44 **Acute suppurative otitis media in children is usually treated with**

a. penicillin V orally
b. amoxycillin orally
c. tetracycline, but only if the child is allergic to penicillin
d. erythromycin if the child is allergic to penicillin
e. gentamicin ear drops

Q.1.45 **The following are types of chronic suppurative otitis media:**

a. Cholesteatoma
b. Tympanosclerosis
c. Tubotympanic disease
d. Adhesive otitis
e. Seromucinous otitis media

For answers see over

Answers

A.1.41 a. T
          b. F
          c. F
          d. F
          e. T

A.1.42 a. T
          b. T
          c. T
          d. F
          e. F

A.1.43 a. T
          b. T
          c. T
          d. F
          e. T

A.1.44 a. T
          b. T—Penicillin or one of the penicillin group are the antibiotics of choice for acute suppurative otitis media.
          c. F—Tetracycline should not be used in children because it stains the teeth.
          d. T
          e. F

A.1.45 a. T
          b. F—Tympanosclerosis is a form of chronic non-suppurative otitis media.
          c. T
          d. F—Adhesive otitis is a non-suppurative condition.
          e. F

Q.1.46 **The following are types of chronic non-suppurative otitis media:**

a. Cholesteatoma
b. Seromucinous otitis media
c. Tympanosclerosis
d. Otosclerosis
e. Adhesive otitis media

Q.1.47 **Tubotympanic chronic suppurative otitis media may**

a. cause deafness
b. produce scanty offensive discharge
c. produce an attic perforation
d. be caused by a labyrinthine fistula
e. rarely occur in children

Q.1.48 **A cholesteatoma**

a. is a middle ear neoplasm
b. is a tumour of the VIIIth nerve
c. is a collection of squamous epithelium in the middle ear cleft
d. may cause intracranial sepsis
e. may cause a lower motor neurone facial paralysis

Q.1.49 **The following are potentially dangerous ear conditions:**

a. Recurrent serous otitis media
b. Tubotympanic type of chronic suppurative otitis media
c. Attico-antral type of chronic suppurative otitis media
d. Central perforation of drumhead
e. Cholesteatoma

Q.1.50 **The following symptom or sign demands prompt operation in attico-antral disease:**

a. Onset of facial paralysis
b. Ipsilateral headache
c. Positive fistula sign
d. Pulsating otorrhoea
e. Onset of vertigo

For answers see over

Answers

A.1.46 a. F
         b. T
         c. T
         d. F—Otosclerosis is a disorder of the otic capsule.
         e. T

A.1.47 a. T
         b. F
         c. F
         d. F
         e. F

A.1.48 a. F—It is effectively a collection of skin within the middle ear.
         b. F
         c. T
         d. T
         e. T

A.1.49 a. F
         b. F
         c. T
         d. F
         e. T

A.1.50 a. T
         b. F—The patient needs urgent investigation in case there is intracranial infection
         c. T
         d. F—Pulsating otorrhoea may merely reflect very active mucosal disease.
         e. F—Unless the fistula sign is positive and/or there is suspicion of a labyrinthine fistula. However, the patient should be investigated urgently.

Q.1.51 **The following are possible complications of chronic suppurative otitis media:**

    a. Meningitis
    b. Extradural abscess
    c. Labyrinthitis
    d. Acute mastoiditis
    e. Acute nephritis

Q.1.52 **An attic retraction pocket**

    a. is a sign of tubotympanic chronic suppurative otitis media
    b. should always be treated by mastoid surgery
    c. is easily seen because an aural polyp is always present
    d. may be difficult to visualise through being obscured by a crust of wax and/or debris
    e. is always associated with a conductive hearing loss

Q.1.53 **A cholesteatoma**

    a. usually causes sensorineural deafness
    b. is associated with a profuse mucopurulent discharge
    c. causes severe earache
    d. usually requires modified radical mastoidectomy
    e. is a premalignant condition

Q.1.54 **An offensive aural discharge may be caused by**

    a. chronic attico-antral disease
    b. otitis externa
    c. both (a) and (b)
    d. tympanosclerosis
    e. carcinoma of the middle ear

Q.1.55 **The operation of choice for a patient with a cholesteatoma is**

    a. radical mastoidectomy
    b. modified radical mastoidectomy
    c. cortical mastoidectomy
    d. myringoplasty
    e. labyrinthectomy

For answers see over

Answers

A.1.51 a. T
          b. T
          c. T
          d. F
          e. F

A.1.52 a. F
          b. F
          c. F—See (d).
          d. T
          e. F—The hearing may be normal.

A.1.53 a. F—But sensorineural deafness may *sometimes* occur.
          b. F—The discharge is usually thin, scanty and offensive.
          c. F—Earache is not a symptom typically associated with cholesteatoma.
          d. T
          e. F

A.1.54 a. T
          b. T
          c. T
          d. F
          e. T

A.1.55 a. F
          b. T
          c. F
          d. F
          e. F

Q.1.56 **A patient who presents with a persistent central perforation which discharges from time to time may be treated by**

    a. long term nasal decongestants
    b. radical mastoidectomy
    c. tympanoplasty
    d. avoidance of swimming and flying
    e. stapedectomy

Q.1.57 **If a patient presents with a persistently discharging central perforation the following aetiological factors should be considered:**

    a. A history of smoking
    b. Allergy to grass pollens
    c. Upper respiratory tract sepsis
    d. HIV infection
    e. Tonsillitis

Q.1.58 **Culture of a chronic suppurative otitis media discharge will grow**

    a. *Staphylococcus aureus*
    b. *Escherichia coli*
    c. *Pseudomonas aeruginosa*
    d. *Proteus mirabilis*
    e. *Streptococcus*

Q.1.59 **Cholesteatoma**

    a. must always be operated on
    b. may cause a serous labyrinthitis
    c. occurs bilaterally in 50%–60% of patients
    d. never occurs in childhood
    e. may occur congenitally

For answers see over

Answers

A.1.56 a. F
          b. F
          c. T
          d. F—Flying does not cause discharge, but swimming may and should be avoided.
          e. F

A.1.57 a. F
          b. F
          c. T
          d. F
          e. F

A.1.58 a. T
          b. T
          c. T
          d. T
          e. F

A.1.59 a. F—It should usually be operated on, but in some circumstances surgery is contraindicated.
          b. T
          c. F
          d. F
          e. T

Q.1.60   Complications of mastoidectomy surgery may include

a. conductive deafness
b. sensorineural deafness
c. facial palsy
d. brain abscess
e. carotico-cavernous fistula

Q.1.61   Modified radical mastoidectomy surgery

a. always produces a dry, safe cavity
b. is always carried out through an endaural incision
c. involves exenterating the mastoid and removing the incus and head of the malleus; it may also include grafting the tympanic membrane
d. will usually cause a deterioration in hearing in the operated ear
e. is the only way of treating a cholesteatoma

Q.1.62   A central tympanic perforation is usually due to

a. tubotympanic chronic suppurative otitis media
b. otomastoiditis
c. cholesteatoma
d. adhesive otitis media
e. trauma

Q.1.63   A perforation of the pars flaccida is usually due to

a. tubotympanitis
b. tympanosclerosis
c. atticoantral disease
d. otosclerosis
e. sinusitis

Q.1.64   Indications for myringoplasty include

a. conductive deafness
b. sensorineural deafness
c. persistent perforation of the membrana tensa
d. recurrent aural discharge through a central perforation
e. attic perforation

For answers see over

Answers

A.1.60 a. T
          b. T—But rare.
          c. T
          d. F
          e. F

A.1.61 a. F—Approximately 20% to 25% of ears operated on remain discharging at some stage.
          b. F—An endaural or postaural approach may be used.
          c. T
          d. F—The relative hearing result depends upon the preoperative level of hearing.
          e. F—There are other surgical methods of treating cholesteatoma.

A.1.62 a. T
          b. T
          c. F
          d. F
          e. F—Trauma *may* cause a central tympanic perforation but is not *usually* the cause.

A.1.63 a. F—The perforation is usually central.
          b. F
          c. T
          d. F
          e. F

A.1.64 a. T—But only if the conductive hearing loss is caused by a central perforation; other pathology may be present within the ear.
          b. F
          c. T
          d. T
          e. F

Q.1.65 Myringoplasty

    a. is 90%–95% successful in closing a perforation of the membrana tensa

    b. should never be carried out if there is a persistent discharge through a central perforation

    c. is contraindicated if a cholesteatoma is suspected

    d. is contraindicated in patients aged over 60

    e. carries a high risk of causing sensorineural deafness

Q.1.66 Tympanoplasty operations

    a. include mastoidectomy and myringoplasty

    b. include myringoplasty and ossicular reconstruction

    c. should only be carried out if the ear has been free of discharge for 4 months

    d. should not be attempted unless bone conduction (i.e., cochlear function) is completely normal in the operated ear

    e. may be indicated in certain cases of otosclerosis

Q.1.67 Most patients with otosclerosis have

    a. a reddish tint to the tympanic membrane

    b. blue sclerae

    c. a retracted drumhead

    d. a normal tympanic membrane

    e. sensorineural deafness

Q.1.68 The pathology in otosclerosis usually involves

    a. fixation of the malleus in the attic region

    b. fixation of the incus in the fossa incudus

    c. fixation of the stapes in the oval window

    d. growth of new bone in (initially rather vascular) specific areas of the temporal bone

    e. obliteration of the round window

For answers see over

Answers

A.1.65 a. T
        b. F—Occasionally it is necessary to proceed with the operation in the presence of a persistent discharge in order to achieve a dry ear
        c. T—Exploration of the ear is required.
        d. F
        e. F

A.1.66 a. F
        b. T—Tympanoplasty equals myringoplasty plus ossiculoplasty.
        c. F
        d. F—But good cochlear function is a prerequisite.
        e. F

A.1.67 a. F—A reddish tint (Schwarz sign) is occasionally seen but only when the disease is very active.
        b. F—But blue sclerae may be seen in Van der Hoeve syndrome (osteogenesis imperfecta with a conductive hearing loss).
        c. F
        d. T
        e. F—But sensorineural deafness may coexist with the conductive hearing loss.

A.1.68 a. F
        b. F
        c. T
        d. T
        e. F

Q.1.69   Otosclerosis

   a. typically affects young to middle aged adults of both sexes
   b. only affects pregnant women
   c. only causes a conductive deafness
   d. causes earache
   e. is never seen in men

Q.1.70   Audiological features of otosclerosis include

   a. a low-frequency conductive deafness
   b. the presence of Carhart's notch
   c. reduced compliance on tympanometry but at normal middle ear pressure
   d. a flat tympanogram
   e. a high tone deafness

Q.1.71   Treatment for otosclerosis may include

   a. a hearing aid
   b. ossiculoplasty
   c. mastoidectomy
   d. stapedectomy
   e. fenestration

Q.1.72   Stapedectomy entails

   a. removal of incus and malleus and replacement with a prosthesis
   b. removal of all or part of the stapes and replacement with a prosthesis
   c. cortical mastoidectomy coupled with removal of all the stapes and replacement with a prosthesis
   d. connecting the incus to the stapes with a prosthesis
   e. an endomeatal approach and reflection of a tympanomeatal flap

For answers see over

Answers

A.1.69   a. T
    b. F—But women with otosclerosis sometimes present in pregnancy.
    c. F—There may sometimes be an associated sensorineural element, and typically a Carhart's notch (a dip in the bone conduction at 2 kHz) is present.
    d. F
    e. F

A.1.70   a. F—The conductive loss is usually relatively flat.
    b. T
    c. T
    d. F
    e. F

A.1.71   a. T
    b. F
    c. F
    d. T
    e. F—The fenestration operation is no longer carried out, having been superseded by stapedectomy.

A.1.72   a. F
    b. T
    c. F
    d. F
    e. T

Q.1.73   The results of stapedectomy

a. are always 100% successful
b. are 85% successful in improving hearing and closing the air-bone gap
c. may sometimes involve development of a severe or profound hearing loss in the operated ear
d. are better in men than women
e. should never be discussed preoperatively with the patient because false hopes may be raised

Q.1.74   Complications of stapedectomy may include

a. sensorineural deafness
b. vertigo
c. meningitis
d. labyrinthitis
e. Ramsay Hunt syndrome

Q.1.75   After stapedectomy the patient must

a. refrain from exercise and exertion for 4–6 weeks
b. use topical ear drops for 1 month
c. not blow his nose for 1 month
d. always wear a hat in cold weather
e. never fly above 10 000 feet

Q.1.76   Adhesive otitis is

a. a synonym for glue ear
b. caused by the introduction of certain dyes into the ear
c. a condition in which fibrous tissue develops within the middle ear, causing adhesions and consequent hearing loss
d. caused by cholesteatoma
e. easily treated with mucolytic agents

For answers see over

Answers

A.1.73 a. F—See (b).
      b. T
      c. T—The risk of a sensorineural hearing loss after stapedectomy is 2% to 5%.
      d. F
      e. F—Morally and medicolegally it is essential to discuss any operation preoperatively when obtaining "informed consent".

A.1.74 a. T
      b. T
      c. F
      d. F—But a labyrinthine fistula may occur postoperatively, causing vertigo.
      e. F

A.1.75 a. T
      b. F
      c. F—But it is wise to avoid nose blowing in the initial postoperative period
      d. F
      e. F

A.1.76 a. F
      b. F
      c. T
      d. F
      e. F

Q.1.77 Tympanosclerosis may cause

    a. sensorineural deafness
    b. mixed deafness
    c. conductive deafness
    d. central perforation of the tympanic membrane
    e. glue ear

Q.1.78 Congenital sensorineural deafness can be caused by

    a. Treacher Collins syndrome
    b. cytomegalovirus infection
    c. prematurity
    d. Waardenburg's syndrome
    e. Down's syndrome

Q.1.79 Total unilateral sensorineural deafness (dead ear) may be caused by

    a. aspirin sensitivity
    b. mumps
    c. trauma
    d. carcinoma of the middle ear
    e. endolymphatic hydrops

Q.1.80 A patient with a dead ear on one side may

    a. be free of symptoms
    b. complain of tinnitus
    c. notice an improvement if treated with steroids for 10 days
    d. be treated with a cochlear implant
    e. need full audiovestibular assessment

Q.1.81 A dead ear on one side in a child aged 5 years may be

    a. missed on school screening tests of hearing
    b. due to infectious parotitis
    c. due to a congenital lesion
    d. ignored
    e. treated with a body-worn hearing aid

For answers see over

Answers

A.1.77 a. F
          b. F
          c. T
          d. F
          e. F—But tympanosclerosis may be associated with secretory otitis and its treatment.

A.1.78 a. F—Treacher Collins syndrome usually produces a conductive hearing loss.
          b. T
          c. T
          d. T
          e. F—Down's syndrome usually produces a conductive hearing loss due to secretory otitis.

A.1.79 a. F—But aspirin may cause a sensorineural deafness.
          b. T
          c. T
          d. T
          e. F—Endolymphatic hydrops rarely cause a dead ear.

A.1.80 a. T—But this is uncommon.
          b. T
          c. F
          d. F—Cochlear implants are essentially reserved for patients with profound bilateral hearing loss.
          e. T

A.1.81 a. T
          b. T
          c. T
          d. F—School teachers and others associated with the child must be made aware of the hearing loss.
          e. F

Q.1.82 **Sudden sensorineural deafness may be caused by**

a. congenital syphilis
b. mumps
c. acoustic neuroma
d. head injury
e. otosclerosis

Q.1.83 **In a patient who presents with sudden sensorineural deafness**

a. referral should be made immediately to an otologist
b. treatment may be with either steroids or a vasodilator regimen, depending on the age of the patient
c. a cerebrovascular accident should always be suspected
d. there will always be a history of a similar episode a few days before
e. if undiagnosed there is a greater risk of a similar occurrence in the other ear

Q.1.84 **Sudden or rapidly progressive unilateral conductive deafness in a young adult**

a. is usually due to otosclerosis
b. may be due to secretory otitis secondary to a nasopharyngeal carcinoma
c. is a common finding in HIV infection
d. is usually due to necrosis of the incus
e. may be safely ignored

Q.1.85 **The typical audiogram of a patient with noise induced hearing loss demonstrates**

a. a 60 dB air–bone gap at 4 kHz
b. a Carhart's notch
c. a dip at 4 kHz with better thresholds at lower and higher frequencies
d. a flat 45 dB loss
e. a dip at 500 Hz on bone conduction

For answers see over

Answers

A.1.82 a. T—But rarely.
          b. T—Typically a unilateral sensorineural hearing loss.
          c. T
          d. T
          e. F

A.1.83 a. T—Referral should be by an immediate telephone call.
          b. T
          c. F
          d. F
          e. F

A.1.84 a. F
          b. T
          c. F
          d. F
          e. F

A.1.85 a. F
          b. F—Carhart's notch is found in otosclerosis and is a dip at 2 kHz in bone conduction.
          c. T
          d. F
          e. F

Q.1.86   Claims for compensation for industrial deafness

a. should be made through a solicitor
b. may be made through the Department of Health for workers in certain occupations
c. will result in loss of pension benefits in later life
d. can be made only if no other cause of deafness is discovered
e. should be initially made through the local police station

Q.1.87   Noise exposure may produce

a. temporary deafness (a temporary threshold shift)
b. permanent deafness (a permanent threshold shift)
c. vertigo
d. otorrhoea
e. tinnitus

Q.1.88   Presbyacusis

a. should always be diagnosed in a patient aged over 65 presenting with deafness
b. usually causes a fluctuating sensorineural deafness
c. should always be treated with a hearing aid
d. may cause a recruiting deafness
e. should be ignored because the patient may have a reduced life expectancy

Q.1.89   Recruitment of hearing

a. is a symptom of acoustic neuroma
b. is usually caused by cochlear hearing loss and may be a symptom of endolymphatic hydrops
c. is the term applied when a patient with a hearing loss finds that suprathreshold sounds appear louder than they actually are
d. should be ignored unless the patient is seeking compensation for industrial deafness
e. may cause difficulties in fitting a hearing aid because only in-the-ear aids may be suitable

For answers see over

Answers

A.1.86 a. T—Claim in law is an action of tort against the employer, and civil legal proceedings should be instituted.
        b. T
        c. F
        d. F
        e. F

A.1.87 a. T
        b. T
        c. T—But very rarely. Extremely loud sound may cause vestibular upset.
        d. F
        e. T

A.1.88 a. F—Other causes of deafness should always be sought.
        b. F—The hearing loss is usually persistent and progressive.
        c. F—A hearing aid is one method of treatment.
        d. T—This may produce problems with fitting a hearing aid and may cause sound intolerance.
        e. F

A.1.89 a. F
        b. T
        c. T
        d. F
        e. F—It may cause difficulty with fitting a hearing aid because the patient has reduced tolerance for loud sound, but in-the-ear aids are no more or less suitable than ear-level aids.

Q.1.90 A patient with an acoustic neuroma will usually demonstrate

a. a recruiting deafness
b. pendular nystagmus
c. absent or reduced responses on caloric testing on the side of the lesion
d. a depressed corneal reflex on the side of the lesion
e. an ipsilateral facial palsy

Q.1.91 Treatment for acoustic neuroma may include

a. radiotherapy
b. intrathecal chemotherapy with cisplatin
c. intracranial exploration and removal
d. observation
e. tarsorrhaphy

Q.1.92 In a man aged 48 presenting with a left sided sensorineural deafness the differential diagnosis should include

a. otosclerosis
b. acoustic neuroma
c. noise deafness
d. congenital syphilis
e. Wegener's granulomatosis

Q.1.93 A patient with acoustic neuroma typically presents with

a. sudden deafness
b. progressive unilateral sensorineural deafness
c. recurrent prolonged bouts of vertigo
d. severe headache, diplopia and blurred vision
e. recurrent meningitis

Q.1.94 Corneal sensitivity testing is a test of

a. oculomotor division of the trigeminal nerve
b. abducens nerve
c. ophthalmic division of the Vth nerve
d. oculomotor division of the trochlear nerve
e. cochleovestibular nerve

For answers see over

Answers

A.1.90 a. F—Recruitment is a sign of a cochlear lesion, not a retro-cochlear one.
      b. F
      c. T
      d. T
      e. F

A.1.91 a. F
      b. F
      c. T
      d. T
      e. F—But tarsorrhaphy may be indicated if a facial palsy develops postoperatively, as commonly occurs in the surgical management of very large acoustic neuromas.

A.1.92 a. F—Otosclerosis normally produces a conductive loss, although exceptionally it may cause sensorineural deafness.
      b. T
      c. F—Industrial noise deafness typically produces a bilateral hearing loss, but patient should be asked about past exposure to noise.
      d. T
      e. F

A.1.93 a. F—But 5% of acoustic neuromas present with sudden sensorineural hearing loss on the affected side.
      b. T
      c. F—Vertiginous spells are uncommon in the natural history of acoustic neuromas.
      d. T—These are all signs of large tumours.
      e. F

A.1.94 a. F
      b. F
      c. T
      d. F
      e. F

Q.1.95 **Corneal sensitivity testing is a test for cranial nerve**

    a. III
    b. IV
    c. V
    d. VI
    e. VII

Q.1.96 **Ménière's disorder is characterised by**

    a. persistent vertigo for several months
    b. episodic vertigo
    c. fluctuating sensorineural hearing loss
    d. conductive deafness
    e. tinnitus

Q.1.97 **Most patients with Ménière's disorder**

    a. need surgical treatment for the vertigo
    b. need surgical treatment to relieve the deafness
    c. suffer also from migraine
    d. are aged over 65
    e. have positive treponemal serology

Q.1.98 **Patients with Ménière's disorder usually show**

    a. a low tone recruiting deafness
    b. caloric abnormalities on vestibular testing
    c. persistent nystagmus to the ipsilateral ear
    d. widening of the internal auditory meatus on tomography of the temporal bone
    e. reduced pressure compliance on tympanometry

Q.1.99 **Treatment of Ménière's disorder**

    a. should always include firm reassurance and full explanation of the nature of the disorder
    b. is usually by destructive labyrinthine surgery
    c. may include salt and fluid deprivation
    d. may be by prescription of betahistine hydrochloride
    e. may cause deterioration in the hearing in the affected ear

For answers see over

Answers

A.1.95 a. F
         b. F
         c. T—It tests the ophthalmic division of the trigeminal nerve.
         d. F
         e. F

A.1.96 a. F—The vertigo occurs usually in discrete bouts, usually lasting many minutes to many hours.
         b. T
         c. T—Typically the hearing loss is initially low tone.
         d. F
         e. T

A.1.97 a. F—But surgery may play a part in the management of a small number of them.
         b. F
         c. F
         d. F
         e. F—But treponemal serology should always be carried out in the investigation of patients with episodic vertigo and a fluctuating or progressive sensorineural hearing loss.

A.1.98 a. T
         b. T
         c. F—Nystagmus is usually seen only during acute spells of vertigo.
         d. F—This may indicate a cerebellopontine angle tumour.
         e. F

A.1.99 a. T—This is the mainstay of any form of treatment for Ménière's disorder.
         b. F—But destructive labyrinthine surgery may be required in a few patients.
         c. T
         d. T—Serc is the trade name of betahistine.
         e. T—Labyrinthectomy will cause a dead ear.

Q.1.100 Surgical treatment of Meniere's disorder may include

a. labyrinthectomy
b. craniotomy and selective vestibular nerve section
c. decompression of the saccus endolymphaticus
d. cochlear drainage into the middle ear
e. insertion of a grommet

Q.1.101 In Ménière's disorder

a. the course is totally unpredictable
b. the course may be predicted on the basis of caloric test results
c. the course can only be predicted if electric response audiometry is carried out
d. stress may contribute to the overall effect
e. the second ear may become involved in up to 50% of patients

Q.1.102 Nystagmus of vestibular origin is usually

a. biphasic and horizontal with a slow and a fast phase
b. pendular
c. suppressed by optic fixation
d. enhanced by optic fixation
e. rotational with a vertical component

Q.1.103 Total labyrinthectomy causes

a. conductive deafness
b. an initial 3rd degree nystagmus to the ipsilateral ear
c. an initial 3rd degree nystagmus to the contralateral ear
d. 1st degree nystagmus to the ipsilateral ear, followed by 2nd
   then 3rd degree nystagmus to that ear
e. sensorineural deafness

For answers see over

Answers

A.1.100 a. T
              b. T
              c. T
              d. F
              e. T—The rationale is far from clear and any beneficial effect may be entirely psychological.

A.1.101 a. T
              b. F
              c. F
              d. T
              e. T

A.1.102 a. T
              b. F
              c. T
              d. F—Nystagmus enhanced by optic fixation suggests a central cause.
              e. F

A.1.103 a. F—It causes a dead ear, i.e., a sensorineural deafness.
              b. F
              c. T
              d. F
              e. T

Q.1.104 3rd degree vestibular nystagmus

a. has the rapid phase in the direction of gaze when looking to one side
b. has the rapid phase in the opposite direction to gaze when looking to one side
c. occurs towards the ipsilateral ear immediately after total labyrinthectomy
d. occurs towards the contralateral ear immediately after total labyrinthectomy
e. is always seen after a successful stapedectomy

Q.1.105 The nystagmus seen in benign paroxysmal positional vertigo

a. is seen only on eye closure
b. is enhanced by abolition of optic fixation
c. is towards the undermost ear with a delay in onset and is fatiguable
d. is away from the undermost ear and is persistent, becoming worse when the patient sits up
e. indicates a brainstem disorder, and long-tract neurological signs may be found on examination

Q.1.106 The extracranial facial nerve

a. leaves the skull via the jugular foramen
b. is deep to the muscles in infants
c. stimulates the stylohyoid muscle
d. runs for approximately 3 cm before bifurcation
e. can branch in eight different ways

Q.1.107 Lower motor neurone facial palsy may be caused by

a. skull fractures
b. viral infections
c. acute ear infections
d. metabolic causes
e. granulomatous disease

For answers see over

Answers

A.1.104   a. F
               b. T
               c. F
               d. T
               e. F

A.1.105   a. F—Nystagmus cannot be seen when the eyes are closed. However, nystagmus may be elicited by the use of electro-nystagmography.
               b. T
               c. T
               d. F—It is directed to the undermost ear, there is a delay in onset, it decays, and it is fatiguable. Any departure from these parameters should alert suspicion of a central cause for the disorder.
               e. F

A.1.106   a. F—Stylomastoid foramen.
               b. F—Subcutaneous.
               c. T
               d. F—2 cm or less.
               e. F—Six types are accepted.

A.1.107   a. T
               b. T
               c. T
               d. T—Acute porphyria.
               e. T—Sarcoidosis/tuberculosis.

Q.1.108 **Investigation of a patient with lower motor neurone facial palsy should include**

a. Schirmer's test
b. stapedius reflex tests on tympanometry
c. Wassermann reaction and other treponemal serology
d. electrogustometry
e. speech audiometry

Q.1.109 **The following disorders may cause lower motor neurone facial palsy:**

a. Acute suppurative otitis media
b. Benign pleomorphic adenoma of the parotid gland
c. Cholesteatoma
d. Herpes zoster virus
e. Sarcoidosis

Q.1.110 **Bell's palsy (idiopathic facial palsy) should always be treated with**

a. prednisone
b. salt and fluid restriction
c. physiotherapy
d. galvanism
e. tarsorrhaphy

Q.1.111 **Facial palsy in children**

a. may be caused by traumatic delivery
b. is usually associated with other congenital defects
c. may be the first sign of hypertension
d. will resolve more quickly with steroid treatment
e. is most commonly idiopathic in origin

Q.1.112 **Bilateral facial palsy may be due to**

a. Guillain-Barré syndrome
b. infectious mononucleosis
c. sarcoidosis
d. diabetes mellitus
e. diabetes insipidus

For answers see over

Answers

A.1.108 a. T
      b. T
      c. F
      d. T
      e. F

A.1.109 a. T
      b. F—A facial palsy with a parotid tumour almost certainly indicates the presence of a malignancy.
      c. T
      d. T—Ramsay Hunt syndrome.
      e. T

A.1.110 a. F—But in some cases steroid therapy may be indicated—for example, in the case of a patient presenting within 48 hours with a total lower motor neurone palsy.
      b. F
      c. F—But physiotherapy may have a marginal effect in maintaining tone in a total lower motor neurone lesion.
      d. F
      e. T—It is essential always to protect the eye, and a lateral tarsorrhaphy may assist in this.

A.1.111 a. T
      b. T
      c. T
      d. F—No evidence, and it may mask a cause.
      e. T—But must be followed up for years.

A.1.112 a. T
      b. T
      c. T
      d. T
      e. F

Q.1.113   Bell's palsy (idiopathic lower motor neurone facial palsy)

a. is self limiting
b. is considered to have a viral aetiology
c. has best prognosis when palsy is incomplete
d. has a good prognosis if movement returns within 21 days
e. is followed by satisfactory functional recovery in more than 95% of cases

Q.1.114   In Ramsay Hunt syndrome (herpes zoster cephalicus)

a. prodromal pain lasting 1 week suggests the diagnosis
b. vesicles in the ear/face are diagnostic
c. dizziness and deafness are rarely seen
d. recurrence of symptoms is common
e. only 60% of patients achieve good recovery of facial function

Q.1.115   In Bell's palsy

a. family history is not important
b. incidence is increased in pregnancy
c. diagnosis is by exclusion
d. long term follow-up is important
e. steroids are always indicated

Q.1.116   Pulsatile tinnitus may be caused by

a. a "hangover"
b. otosclerosis
c. carotid aneurysms and carotico-cavernous fistula
d. glomus jugulare tumours
e. noise exposure

Q.1.117   A glomus jugulare tumour is

a. a vascular neoplasm usually situated at the jugular foramen
b. a lesion on the base of the tongue
c. a cause of pulsatile tinnitus
d. a malignant intracranial tumour extending through the jugular foramen
e. may produce physical signs associated with cranial nerves IX, X and XI

For answers see over

Answers

A.1.113   a. T
          b. T
          c. T
          d. T
          e. F—Only 80% have acceptable recovery.

A.1.114   a. T
          b. T
          c. T
          d. F—Bell's palsy has a recurrence risk of 12% .
          e. T

A.1.115   a. F
          b. T
          c. T
          d. T
          e. F—Should seldom be indicated; may delay or mask the real cause of the palsy.

A.1.116   a. F
          b. F
          c. T
          d. T
          e. F

A.1.117   a. T
          b. F
          c. T
          d. F—It is benign.
          e. T

Q.1.118 **The treatment for glomus jugulare tumours may include**

a. ligation of the internal jugular vein
b. radiotherapy
c. surgical removal
d. vascular embolisation with Gelfoam
e. watchful waiting

Q.1.119 **Malignant tumours of the middle ear are associated with**

a. radiotherapy
b. chronic suppurative otitis media
c. chemical irritation
d. psoriatic otitis externa
e. furunculosis

Q.1.120 **Malignant tumours of the middle ear**

a. should be suspected when pain is severe
b. may represent a metastasis
c. are always suitable for curative treatment
d. are frequently squamous cell carcinoma
e. have a good 5-year survival

Q.1.121 **In-the-ear hearing aids**

a. should always be offered to women with a hearing loss because they are more acceptable cosmetically
b. are available in the UK through the National Health Service
c. are best for babies and young children because they are more difficult to remove
d. have a limited usefulness because of relatively low gain and output
e. may be worn for any water sports

For answers see over

Answers

A.1.118 a. F
          b. T
          c. T
          d. T
          e. T

A.1.119 a. T
          b. T
          c. F
          d. F
          e. F

A.1.120 a. T
          b. T
          c. F
          d. T
          e. F

A.1.121 a. F—Paradoxically they are perhaps more appropriate for men, since many women can conceal a hearing aid with a suitable hair style.
          b. F
          c. F
          d. T
          e. F

Q.1.122   Bone conductor hearing aids should be used

   a. never
   b. in patients with conductive deafness
   c. in patients with bilateral meatal atresia
   d. in bilateral intractable otitis externa
   e. in patients with presbyacusis

Q.1.123   For a baby with severe or profound sensorineural deafness

   a. hearing aids should not be prescribed under age 18 months
   b. hearing aids should not be prescribed under age 12 months
   c. early detection and rehabilitation are essential
   d. the most appropriate hearing aid is a bone conductor aid
   e. the provision of information about available services is subject to statutory requirements

Q.1.124   Cochlear implants

   a. are useless
   b. provide normal hearing
   c. enable the user to detect sound, but hearing will not be normal
   d. may be offered to anyone with severe or profound hearing loss
   e. should never be fitted to children aged under 10 years

For answers see over

Answers

A.1.122   a. F
  b. F—However, if the conductive loss is due to chronic sup-
     purative otitis media with a persistent discharge any insert aid
     may be quite inappropriate and a bone conductor aid should
     be used.
  c. T
  d. T
  e. F

A.1.123   a. F—As soon as the diagnosis is established, an aid should be
     prescribed in order to avoid auditory deprivation.
  b. F
  c. T
  d. F
  e. T

A.1.124   a. F—However, cochlear implants do not produce normal
     hearing but essentially produce an awareness of sound.
  b. F
  c. T
  d. F—The patient needs to be investigated fully, both physically
     and psychologically; a cochlear implant is suitable only for
     patients with total loss of hearing due to cochlear pathology.
  e. F

2. Nose

Q.2.1 Nasal mucus

a. helps with humidification of inspired air
b. protects the normal nasal tissue
c. is normally sterile
d. shows yellow discoloration when infected
e. has a high content of IgE and IgA

Q.2.2 Adenoids

a. are mucus secreting organs
b. are located in the roof of the nose
c. can cause snoring as they move
d. are involved in immune reactions
e. are a common source of chronic sepsis

Q.2.3 Nasal resistance

a. can be altered by atmospheric conditions
b. is maximal posteriorly
c. is controlled by the parasympathetic nerve
d. is difficult to measure
e. is increased by a crooked septum

Q.2.4 Regarding nasal anatomy:

a. The paranasal sinuses are ectodermal in origin
b. The frontal sinus is present at birth
c. The nasolacrimal duct opens below the middle turbinate
d. A crooked nasal septum is uncommon
e. Some of the blood supply to the nose is by the internal carotid artery

Q.2.5 Nasal swabbing in symptom free patients may reveal

a. *Staphylococcus aureus*
b. *Streptococcus β* haemolytic type
c. *Haemophilus influenzae*
d. no organisms
e. coagulase positive *Streptococcus*

For answers see over

Answers

A.2.1 a. T
      b. T
      c. F
      d. F—Eosinophils can produce yellow mucus (an allergic reaction).
      e. T

A.2.2 a. F—Lymphoid tissue.
      b. F—They are located in the posterosuperior area of the naso-pharynx.
      c. F—If the adenoids moved so would the head !
      d. T
      e. F

A.2.3 a. T
      b. F—Resistance is maximal in the nasal vestibule and anterior end of the turbinates.
      c. F—It is controlled by sympathetic activity.
      d. T—Rhinomanometry is the only method currently available.
      e. T—Correction will improve symptoms.

A.2.4 a. T
      b. F—It can be recognised on X-ray by about age 6 years.
      c. F—It opens anteriorly below the inferior turbinate.
      d. F—Reportedly found in more than 80% of the population.
      e. T—By the anterior and posterior ethmoidal arteries.

A.2.5 a. T
      b. F
      c. F
      d. T
      e. F—It is the most common pathogen of the nasal vestibule.

Q.2.6 Olfactory function (smell)

a. is controlled by non-myelinated nerves
b. is little affected by age
c. when enhanced indicates pathology
d. is commonly affected by nasal polyps
e. is not affected by head injuries to the occipital area

Q.2.7 Congenital nasal mass lesions

a. most commonly present in young adults
b. may contain "glial" tissue
c. commonly present (as nasal polyps) in children
d. may communicate with the meninges
e. tend to recur if ectodermal

Q.2.8 Congenital choanal atresia

a. has an incidence of 1 in 10 000 live births
b. if unilateral may remain undiagnosed
c. results from a membranous defect
d. requires surgical management if bilateral
e. is associated with other congenital defects

Q.2.9 Regarding a blocked nose/nasal obstruction in infancy:

a. Septal deviation is uncommon at birth
b. Foreign bodies may need removal using general anaesthesia
c. It is essential to test for catheter patency of nasal passages
d. Congenital nasal masses are frequently found at birth
e. Antibiotics are the treatment of choice

Q.2.10 Foreign bodies in the nose

a. are most frequently found in the left nostril
b. are frequently found in children and the mentally retarded
c. often present as a nose bleed
d. are in most cases diagnosed by X-ray
e. can usually be removed in the clinic

For answers see over

Answers

A.2.6 a. T
        b. F—Loss increases with age.
        c. F—Hyperosmia is rarely pathological.
        d. T—Removal may help, but no guarantee should be given.
        e. F—More likely than with frontal trauma.

A.2.7 a. F—The majority of cases present by age 5 years.
        b. T—They may also present extranasally glioma.
        c. F—Polyps are seldom seen in children.
        d. T—All encephalocoeles, 10% of gliomas and some dermoids communicate with the meninges.
        e. T—Infection makes surgical excision difficult.

A.2.8 a. F—The incidence is 1 in 8000 live births.
        b. T—It causes unilateral discharge in adulthood.
        c. F—90% of defects are bony.
        d. T—Usually within the first week of life.
        e. T—60% of cases are associated with other defects.

A.2.9 a. F—50%
        b. T
        c. T
        d. F
        e. F—They are seldom helpful in infancy.

A.2.10 a. F—They are usually located in the right nostril.
        b. T
        c. F—They usually present as a unilateral foetid discharge.
        d. F—The majority are diagnosed by inspection.
        e. T—But uncooperative patients need general anaesthesia.

Q.2.11 In a child with a runny nose

a. a normal sinus X-ray excludes sinusitis
b. removal of enlarged adenoids is helpful
c. adenoidectomy will cure nocturnal coughing
d. surgery seldom effects a cure
e. if symptoms are due to allergic rhinitis the best treatment is avoidance of allergens

Q.2.12 In cystic fibrosis

a. nasal symptoms are present in more than 50% of cases
b. nasal polyps may be present
c. the radiological appearance of the sinuses is normal
d. nasal symptoms can be managed surgically
e. sinusitis predisposes to glue ear

Q.2.13 Nose bleeds in children

a. are seldom serious
b. are usually from a visible site
c. are always cured by appropriate treatment
d. can be reduced in frequency by local antiseptic ointment
e. are often due to "picking", and this needs to be excluded before treatment

Q.2.14 Regarding nose bleeds in children:

a. Chronic sinusitis needs to be ruled out in recurrent cases
b. Measles may precipitate nose bleeds
c. Surgery is indicated in resistant cases
d. They may be the initial presentation of angiofibromas in girls
e. Bleeding usually arises from Little's area

Q.2.15 Nasal vestibulitis

a. may be secondary to furunculosis
b. is a trivial complaint
c. should always be treated with systemic antibiotics
d. if unilateral, should suggest a foreign body
e. if chronic, due to sinusitis, may cause bilateral excoriation

For answers see over

Answers

A.2.11   a. F
         b. T—Improves air movement through the nasal cavity.
         c. F—There is currently no evidence.
         d. T
         e. T

A.2.12   a. F—Only 30% approximately have nasal symptoms.
         b. T—In less than 10% they may be the first sign.
         c. F—Abnormal in almost all patients.
         d. F—Surgery is of little help in the long term.
         e. F—The risk is no greater than in the general population.

A.2.13   a. T
         b. T
         c. F
         d. T
         e. T

A.2.14   a. T
         b. T
         c. T—Cautery under either local or general anaesthetic.
         d. F—A disease of young boys.
         e. T—Anterior end of nasal septum.

A.2.15   a. T
         b. F—It may progress to cavernous sinus thrombosis.
         c. F—Local antibiotic cream is usually effective.
         d. T
         e. T—Treatment should be directed at the sinusitis.

Q.2.16 **A patient with complete anosmia should respond to inhalation of**

a. coffee
b. chocolate
c. oil of lemon
d. ammonia
e. tobacco

Q.2.17 **Olfactory sensibility**

a. always returns after bilateral polypectomy
b. provides the "flavour" component to taste
c. is unaffected by total laryngectomy
d. is lost after fracture of the cribriform plate
e. fatigues quickly

Q.2.18 **The paranasal sinuses**

a. drain mainly into the middle meatus
b. drain mainly into the inferior meatus
c. are lined with transitional epithelium
d. may contain olfactory epithelium
e. contain expired air

Q.2.19 **Causes of nose bleeds include**

a. fingers
b. upper respiratory tract infections
c. snuff
d. nasal polyps
e. trauma

Q.2.20 **Regarding nasal trauma:**

a. More than 50% need no treatment
b. X-rays are essential in all nasal fractures
c. Reduction with splintage may reduce cosmetic deformity
d. Traumatic swelling should be reduced by ice packs before assessment
e. Direct trauma is uncommon

For answers see over

Answers

A.2.16 a. F
          b. F
          c. F
          d. T—Ammonia stimulates the sensory endings of the Vth nerve.
          e. F

A.2.17 a. F
          b. T
          c. F
          d. T
          e. T

A.2.18 a. T
          b. F
          c. F
          d. F
          e. T

A.2.19 a. T
          b. T
          c. F
          d. F
          e. T

A.2.20 a. T
          b. F—X-rays are indicated when mid-facial fractures also are suspected.
          c. T
          d. F—Review in 5 days.
          e. F—Usually mid-facial fractures.

Q.2.21   Nasal trauma

a. is best assessed at 24 hours
b. is best assessed at 5 days
c. is best assessed at 5 weeks
d. is usually associated with septal haematoma
e. often requires no treatment

Q.2.22   Unilateral nasal discharge may be due to

a. foreign body
b. tumour
c. encephalocoele
d. large adenoids
e. septal perforation

Q.2.23   Regarding recurrent spontaneous nose bleeds:

a. The diagnosis is epistaxis
b. Underlying systemic disease needs to be looked for
c. Most arise from the anterior septal area
d. Cautery is effective in the acute phase
e. Local pressure for 5 minutes will stop venous haemorrhage

Q.2.24   Epistaxis in the elderly

a. is associated with atherosclerosis
b. is associated with hypertension
c. in many cases arises from an invisible bleeding point
d. can be arrested by intranasal packing
e. may need arterial ligation if resistant

Q.2.25   Nasal septal deviation

a. seldom causes symptoms
b. always causes unilateral nasal obstruction
c. may cause pain
d. always requires surgical correction
e. requires correction under a general anaesthetic

For answers see over

Answers

A.2.21 a. F
        b. T
        c. F
        d. F—But needs to be excluded at initial presentation.
        e. T

A.2.22 a. T
        b. T
        c. T
        d. F
        e. F

A.2.23 a. F—Epistaxis is the medical term for nose bleeds.
        b. T
        c. T
        d. T
        e. T

A.2.24 a. T—Bleeds are more profuse in patients with atherosclerosis.
        b. F—Usually bleeds are more severe, but hypertension is not the cause of the bleeds.
        c. T
        d. T—In the majority of cases.
        e. F—Most will need correction of septal deformity with packing.

A.2.25 a. T
        b. F—Usually bilateral.
        c. F
        d. F—Only if symptomatic.
        e. F—Can be performed under local anaesthetic.

Q.2.26 **Nasal septal trauma (soft tissue trauma)**

a. can result in septal haematoma
b. may require X-ray for diagnosis of septal haematoma
c. does not usually require treatment
d. can result in deformity of the nose
e. rarely results in septal abscess

Q.2.27 **Nasal packing to control a nose bleed**

a. rarely needs local anaesthetic
b. should be used in conjunction with an antiseptic if required for longer than 48 hours
c. requires antibiotic cover when used for longer than 48 hours
d. may be achieved with a Foley catheter
e. is used for most patients with epistaxis

Q.2.28 **Nasal septal surgery**

a. is abbreviated to NSS
b. rarely leads to septal perforation
c. may be followed by persistent nasal obstruction
d. is usually part of corrective cosmetic surgery
e. is indicated in all patients with symptoms

Q.2.29 **An alternative to straightening of a crooked septum is**

a. resection of the turbinates
b. septal dermoplasty
c. lateral rhinotomy
d. rhinoplasty
e. septoplasty

Q.2.30 **Septal perforation can be caused by**

a. cocaine addiction
b. septal surgery
c. chromium exposure
d. malignant disease
e. "picking"

For answers see over

Answers

A.2.26 a. T
           b. F—By inspection.
           c. F
           d. T
           e. F—It may occur secondarily to a septal haematoma.

A.2.27 a. T
           b. F
           c. T
           d. T
           e. T—For those who attend hospital.

A.2.28 a. F—The operation is submucous resection of the nasal septum (SMR).
           b. F—It is the most frequent cause of septal perforation.
           c. T—Because of inadequate surgery, perforation, or adhesions.
           d. T
           e. F—Should not be performed in children.

A.2.29 a. T
           b. F—septal dermoplasty is performed for septal telangiectasia.
           c. F—lateral rhinotomy is performed for nasal tumours.
           d. F—rhinoplasty implies only surgery to the nasal skeleton.
           e. T—septoplasty removes only the crooked cartilage and leaves the straight cartilage.

A.2.30 a. T
           b. T
           c. T
           d. T
           e. T

Q.2.31 **Symptoms of septal perforation may include**

a. "whistling"
b. bleeding/crusting
c. nasal discharge
d. obstruction
e. pain

Q.2.32 **Investigation and management of 'sinusitis' must include**

a. good symptom details
b. X-rays
c. examination of the nose
d. family history
e. social habits

Q.2.33 **The following may predispose to sinusitis:**

a. Hypertrophy of the superior turbinate
b. Adenoidal hypertrophy in children
c. Marked deviation of the nasal septum
d. Honeymoon rhinitis
e. Enlarged middle turbinate

Q.2.34 **"Rhinitis" may be classified as**

a. allergic
b. infective
c. iatrogenic
d. familial
e. environmental

Q.2.35 **Nasal congestion is commoner in women because**

a. they are more prone to anxiety reactions
b. they are subject to cyclical hormonal variations
c. pregnancy increases susceptibility
d. the progesterone contraceptive pill increases susceptibility
e. myxoedema increases susceptibility and is commoner in women

For answers see over

Answers

A.2.31 a. T
        b. T
        c. F
        d. T
        e. F

A.2.32 a. T
        b. F
        c. T
        d. F
        e. T

A.2.33 a. F
        b. T
        c. T
        d. F
        e. T

A.2.34 a. T
        b. T
        c. T—Including self inflicted.
        d. T—Very rare.
        e. F—Usually called allergic.

A.2.35 a. F
        b. T
        c. T
        d. F—Only with high-oestrogen contraceptive pill.
        e. T

Q.2.36   Allergic rhinitis

    a. is an IgE mediated hypersensitivity
    b. is characterised by sneezing
    c. is more common in children than adults
    d. affects more than 25% of the population
    e. is most commonly caused by grass pollen

Q.2.37   Patients with "aspirin intolerance" have a higher than normal risk of developing

    a. nasal polyps
    b. asthma
    c. sinusitis
    d. hyperplastic sinuses
    e. positive allergic skin tests

Q.2.38   In allergic rhinitis desensitisation

    a. is indicated in all patients
    b. may result in anaphylaxis and possibly death
    c. can usually relieve symptoms after a single treatment
    d. is given by intramuscular injection
    e. to grass and pollen is unpredictable.

Q.2.39   The enlarged inferior turbinate may clinically be mistaken for

    a. nasal polyp
    b. septal deviation
    c. encephalocoele
    d. septal abscess
    e. foreign body

Q.2.40   The enlarged inferior turbinate

    a. may present as nasal obstruction
    b. may result from a septal deformity
    c. occasionally has a "blue" colour
    d. can be treated symptomatically with surgery
    e. causes a bad smell in the nose

For answers see over

Answers

A.2.36 a. T
         b. F—sneezing with obstruction and discharge.
         c. F
         d. F—10%–15%.
         e. T

A.2.37 a. T
         b. T
         c. F
         d. T
         e. F—Usually negative skin tests.

A.2.38 a. F
         b. T—Should only be carried out in hospital.
         c. F—Frequently needs to be repeated.
         d. F—Subcutaneously only.
         e. F—Usually effective.

A.2.39 a. T
         b. T
         c. F—However, an encephalocoele may look like a polyp.
         d. F—Septal abscesses are usually seen on both sides.
         e. F—A good history will usually help.

A.2.40 a. T
         b. T
         c. T
         d. T
         e. F

Q.2.41 **Acute-onset of nasal discharge with pain**

a. may be viral in origin
b. may be bacterial in origin
c. has no known effective treatment
d. can be quickly cured with antibiotics
e. is more common in winter because rhinoviruses are prevalent

Q.2.42 **The pain of "sinusitis" may be**

a. migraine
b. caused by periapical abscess
c. psychogenic
d. caused by depressive illness
e. tic douloureux

Q.2.43 **The bacteria most frequently causing acute sinusitis include**

a. *Streptococcus pneumoniae*
b. *Staphylococcus aureus*
c. *Haemophilus influenzae*
d. *Neisseria catarrhalis*
e. Mixed organisms

Q.2.44 **The following clinical symptoms if present in acute sinusitis require hospital referral:**

a. Pain
b. Vomiting
c. Nominal aphasia
d. Drowsiness
e. Purulent nasal discharge

Q.2.45 **Relief of pain in acute sinusitis may be achieved with**

a. antibiotics
b. decongestants
c. analgesics
d. sinus "wash out"
e. local heat

For answers see over

Answers

A.2.41 a. T
          b. T
          c. T
          d. F
          e. F

A.2.42 a. T
          b. T
          c. T
          d. T
          e. T

A.2.43 a. T
          b. F
          c. T
          d. F—Rarely.
          e. T

A.2.44 a. F
          b. T
          c. T
          d. T
          e. F

A.2.45 a. F
          b. F
          c. T
          d. T
          e. T

Q.2.46 **The treatment of acute sinusitis should include**

a. analgesics
b. local vasoconstrictor drops
c. antibiotics
d. hospital referral
e. hypnotics

Q.2.47 **The following signs on X-ray are consistent with acute sinusitis:**

a. Opaque maxillary antrum
b. Air/fluid level
c. Bone destruction
d. Mucosal thickening
e. Normal pictures

Q.2.48 **The radiological sign of air/fluid level in the maxillary antrum is consistent with a diagnosis of**

a. cerebrospinal leak
b. sinusitis
c. trauma
d. tumour
e. nothing pathological

Q.2.49 **Maxillary sinusitis may be caused by infection of the following teeth:**

a. "Wisdom"
b. Canine
c. Second premolar
d. Incisor
e. First molar

For answers see over

Answers

A.2.46 a. T
          b. T
          c. T
          d. F
          e. F

A.2.47 a. T
          b. T
          c. F
          d. T
          e. T

A.2.48 a. T
          b. T
          c. T
          d. F
          e. T

A.2.49 a. F
          b. F
          c. F
          d. F
          e. T

Q.2.50 Early referral is indicated in patients who complain of head-ache associated with

   a. interruption of nocturnal sleep
   b. relief by a period of sleep
   c. vomiting
   d. onset of neck stiffness
   e. pressure "band like" tension of the head

Q.2.51 Regarding sinusitis and the dental surgeon:

   a. Caries of the canine teeth may cause sinusitis
   b. Recent dental surgery may cause sinusitis
   c. A normal occlusal film is reassuring
   d. A creamy antral aspirate suggests dental aetiology
   e. Facial fractures in the past may be the cause.

Q.2.52 In chronic sinusitis

   a. cure is common
   b. a week's course of antibiotics is adequate
   c. nasal discharge is helped by an antral lavage
   d. pain is easily relieved
   e. nasal discharge can be helped by local medications

Q.2.53 The diagnosis of chronic sinusitis is suggested by

   a. nasal congestion
   b. recurrent cheek pain
   c. nasal obstruction with discharge
   d. nasal pain with discharge
   e. nasal discharge with obstruction and pain

Q.2.54 The aims of surgical management of chronic sinusitis are to

   a. improve drainage of the sinuses
   b. alleviate pain
   c. prevent intracranial sepsis
   d. return the antral mucosa to normal
   e. allow aeration of the sinuses

For answers see over

Answers

A.2.50 a. T—Raised intracranial pressure.
        b. F—Usually cluster headaches or migraine.
        c. T—Meningeal irritation.
        d. T—Subarachnoid haemorrhage.
        e. F—Tension headaches.

A.2.51 a. F
        b. T
        c. F
        d. T—Many patients have a bad smell in the nose
        e. T

A.2.52 a. F
        b. F—Usually needed for weeks if not months.
        c. T
        d. F
        e. T

A.2.53 a. T
        b. F—? Dental.
        c. T
        d. F
        e. T

A.2.54 a. T
        b. F
        c. T
        d. F
        e. T

Q.2.55 In chronic pansinusitis

a. only the frontal sinuses are involved
b. the maxillary sinus is the dominant sinus
c. nasal polyps are common
d. bronchiectasis may be associated
e. surgical management will always lead to cure

Q.2.56 Complications of sinusitis may include

a. mucocoele
b. laryngitis
c. blindness
d. death
e. deafness

Q.2.57 Complications of sinusitis include

a. subdural abscess
b. frontal lobe abscess
c. temporal lobe abscess
d. cerebellar abscess
e. extradural abscess

Q.2.58 The Caldwell Luc approach to the maxillary sinus (radical antrotomy)

a. may be useful in chronic maxillary sinusitis
b. leaves a permanent oroantral fistula
c. may be used in suspected malignancy
d. has a place in the control of arterial epistaxis
e. is used to remove nasal polyps

Q.2.59 The incidence of chronic suppurative sinusitis is increased in

a. chronic bronchitis
b. bronchiectasis
c. nasal polyposis
d. Kartagener's syndrome
e. secretory otitis media

For answers see over

Answers

A.2.55
  a. F
  b. T
  c. T
  d. T
  e. F—But it may sometimes be effective.

A.2.56
  a. T
  b. T
  c. T
  d. T
  e. F

A.2.57
  a. T
  b. T
  c. F—Usually otogenic abscess.
  d. F
  e. T

A.2.58
  a. T
  b. F
  c. F—Should not be used.
  d. T—To approach the sphenopalatine artery.
  e. F

A.2.59
  a. F
  b. T
  c. T
  d. T
  e. F

Q.2.60 **Facial swelling may be caused by**

    a. cancer of the maxillary sinus
    b. sinusitis
    c. cutaneous inflammation
    d. dental abscess
    e. mumps

Q.2.61 **The following can usually be differentiated on plain film radiographs:**

    a. Acute and chronic sinusitis
    b. Frontal sinus mucocoele and carcinoma
    c. Posterior choanal polyps and adenoidal enlargement
    d. Benign papilloma and carcinoma of the larynx
    e. Mastoid cholesteatoma and carcinoma

Q.2.62 **Proof puncture (antral wash out)**

    a. is a needlessly punishing treatment
    b. includes aspiration of the antral contents
    c. can be uncomfortable
    d. may result in "false puncture"
    e. may result in bleeding

Q.2.63 **Presenting symptoms suggestive of nasal polyps include**

    a. nasal obstruction
    b. pain
    c. bloody discharge
    d. anosmia
    e. rhinorrhoea

Q.2.64 **Nasal polyps**

    a. may arise from the ethmoid sinus
    b. can be seen in the inferior meatus
    c. may be premalignant
    d. are usually unilateral
    e. are common in children

For answers see over

Answers

A.2.60   a. T
   b. F
   c. T
   d. T
   e. F

A.2.61   a. F
   b. F
   c. T
   d. F
   e. F

A.2.62   a. F
   b. T
   c. T—Needs adequate explanation before the procedure.
   d. T—Puncture into the local soft tissues may occur.
   e. T—For up to 12 hours.

A.2.63   a. T
   b. F
   c. F—Suggests a more sinister condition.
   d. T
   e. T

A.2.64   a. T
   b. F—Middle meatus below the middle turbinate.
   c. F
   d. F—Most frequently bilateral.
   e. F—Only in cystic fibrosis

Q.2.65 **Histologically, unilateral nasal "polyp" may be**

a. benign inflammatory
b. malignant melanoma
c. transitional-cell papilloma
d. metastatic malignant disease
e. meningioma

Q.2.66 **In patients who present with crusting, epistaxis and nasal obstruction may be the diagnosis indicated**

a. syphilis
b. diabetes mellitus
c. tuberculosis
d. leprosy
e. hypertension

Q.2.67 **Chronic atrophic rhinitis**

a. starts at puberty
b. is more common in females
c. has a well-documented aetiology
d. may be caused by syphilis
e. can be improved symptomatically with nasal douching

Q.2.68 **Regarding nasal polyps:**

a. Skin tests are usually positive
b. Patients with atopia and asthma present earlier
c. Women are more commonly affected
d. Coloured people are rarely affected
e. Medical management is a waste of time

Q.2.69 **Antrochoanal polyp**

a. arises from the ethmoid sinus
b. can usually be seen on anterior rhinoscopy
c. usually causes unilateral symptoms
d. is thought to have an infective aetiology
e. can be managed symptomatically with polypectomy

For answers see over

Answers

A.2.65 a. T
      b. T—Rare.
      c. T
      d. F
      e. T

A.2.66 a. T
      b. F
      c. T
      d. T
      e. F

A.2.67 a. T
      b. T
      c. F—Aetiology is unknown.
      d. F—It is a specific disease.
      e. T—Daily douching with warm saline followed by glucose/ glycerine drops.

A.2.68 a. F—No more commonly than in the general population.
      b. F
      c. F—Four times as common in men.
      d. F—No racial differences.
      e. F—Steroid drops are usually effective.

A.2.69 a. F—The maxillary antrum.
      b. F—Posterior rhinoscopy.
      c. T
      d. F—Aetiology unknown.
      e. F—Usually requires Caldwell Luc approach.

Q.2.70 **The Caldwell Luc approach to the maxillary sinus**

    a. carries a risk of oroantral fistula
    b. uncommonly causes paraesthesia of the lip
    c. requires removal of only the diseased mucosa
    d. is through the nose
    e. can cure chronic sinus disease

Q.2.71 **Surgical management of nasal polyps**

    a. is inadequate if polyps recur
    b. should be followed by medical management postoperatively
    c. by an intranasal approach may damage the eye
    d. by an external approach ensures cure
    e. is indicated only after failed medical management

Q.2.72 **A patient with symptoms persisting after a Caldwell Luc operation should be investigated with**

    a. antroscopy
    b. clinical examination
    c. sinus X-rays
    d. computed tomography
    e. sinus irrigation

Q.2.73 **A patient with rhinitis due to defective mucociliary clearance may also have symptoms of**

    a. deafness
    b. chronic cough
    c. infertility
    d. diarrhoea
    e. dysphagia

Q.2.74 **In rhinitis medicamentosa (iatrogenic rhinitis)**

    a. the cause is usually abuse of topical nasal decongestants
    b. rebound is rare
    c. sensations of burning and dryness can be intolerable
    d. tachyphylaxis is common
    e. treatment is by cessation of topical decongestants

For answers see over

Answers

A.2.70 a. T
  b. F—Common enough for every patient to be warned before operation.
  c. F—Recurrence of symptoms is inevitable unless complete mucosal clearance is carried out.
  d. F—Approach is under the upper lip.
  e. T

A.2.71 a. F—Recurrence is a feature of the disease.
  b. T
  c. T
  d. F
  e. T

A.2.72 a. T
  b. F—Usually unhelpful.
  c. F—The sinus will be opaque.
  d. T
  e. T

A.2.73 a. T
  b. T
  c. T
  d. F
  e. F

A.2.74 a. T
  b. F—Secondary hyperaemia (rebound) occurs a few hours after administration.
  c. T
  d. T—Increasing quantities of the drug are required to elicit a given response.
  e. T

Q.2.75 **Skin testing in allergic rhinitis**

a. is essential for making the diagnosis.
b. is not affected by systemic steroid treatment
c. should be done on prepared skin only
d. can be affected by some H2 antagonist drugs
e. produces a maximal wheal within 5 minutes

Q.2.76 **Investigation of nasal symptoms may include**

a. nasal bacteriological swab
b. RAST testing
c. biochemistry profile
d. ultrasound
e. transillumination

Q.2.77 **The following nasal symptoms may suggest a possible tumour:**

a. Epiphora
b. Epistaxis
c. Sneezing
d. Pain
e. Anaesthesia of the upper lip

Q.2.78 **Transitional papillomata of the nose**

a. are usually bilateral
b. occur only in the elderly
c. are cured with radiotherapy
d. need not be followed up after 5 years
e. carry a high risk of malignancy

Q.2.79 **Complications following tonsillectomy include**

a. increased nasality of speech
b. death
c. persistent sore throat
d. ear infections
e. regrowth of tonsils

For answers see over

Answers

A.2.75   a.   F—History is the mainstay
          b.   T
          c.   F
          d.   T—The drugs need to be stopped some 4 weeks before tests.
          e.   F—Usually takes 15 minutes.

A.2.76   a.   T
          b.   T—Allergy test.
          c.   F
          d.   T
          e.   T—However, no longer used.

A.2.77   a.   T
          b.   F—Usually blood tinged nasal discharge more suggestive.
          c.   F
          d.   T—However, usually a late sign.
          e.   T—Involvement of the inferior orbital nerve.

A.2.78   a.   F—Unilateral.
          b.   F—Any age, usually five times more common in men.
          c.   F—Radical surgical excision is required.
          d.   F—Lifelong follow-up once diagnosed.
          e.   F—2%–5% risk.

A.2.79   a.   T
          b.   T
          c.   T—Depending on the accuracy of the preoperative diagnosis.
          d.   F—Usually referred earache rather than infective disease.
          e.   F—Usually indicates inadequate primary surgery.

Q.2.80 Osteoma of the paranasal sinuses

a. is diagnosed by radiology
b. is usually asymptomatic
c. is most frequently found in the ethmoid sinus
d. can displace the globe
e. presents with symptoms of sinus obstruction

Q.2.81 Regarding neoplasms of the nasal vestibule:

a. They are always malignant
b. Basal cell carcinomas are painful
c. Longstanding ulceration suggests squamous cancer
d. Treatment is indicated by appearances
e. Treatment usually includes radiotherapy

Q.2.82 Malignant nasal tumours

a. account for only 3% of all nasal tumours recorded
b. are frequently diagnosed as "sinusitis"
c. have a good prognosis
d. are squamous carcinoma in 80% of cases
e. are especially common in woodworkers

Q.2.83 Malignant nasal tumours

a. are frequently unsuitable for curative treatment
b. are usually treated with radiotherapy
c. seldom involve the eye
d. are treated surgically, but for palliation of symptoms only
e. carry a 5 year survival of over 30%.

Q.2.84 Wegener's granulomatosis

a. has a viral aetiology
b. is granulomatous disease of the nose, lung and kidney
c. is difficult to diagnose histologically
d. is treated with local radiotherapy
e. is inevitably fatal

For answers see over

Answers

A.2.80 a. T
b. T—The majority.
c. F—Frontal sinus.
d. T
e. T

A.2.81 a. F—Most common lesion is papilloma.
b. F—Usually painless.
c. F—Squamous carcinoma usually rapid in onset.
d. F—Biopsy confirmation mandatory before treatment.
e. T

A.2.82 a. F—Less than 1%.
b. T
c. F—Poor because of delayed accurate diagnosis.
d. T
e. T—Adenocarcinoma of the ethmoid.

A.2.83 a. T
b. T—However, may not be given with curative intent.
c. F
d. F—Usually combined with radiotherapy for cure.
e. F—Less than 30%.

A.2.84 a. F—Aetiology unknown.
b. T
c. T—If diagnosis is suspected multiple repeated biopsies may be required to confirm diagnosis.
d. F—Chemotherapy.
e. F—Uncommon; death usually from renal failure.

Q.2.85 The initial symptoms/signs of cancer of the nasopharynx may be

a. facial pain
b. epistaxis
c. nasal obstruction
d. serous otitis media
e. diplopia

Q.2.86 Patients who receive radiotherapy to the nasopharynx may years later develop

a. choanal polyps
b. atrophic rhinitis
c. loss of taste
d. nasopharyngeal cancer
e. neurogenic tumours of the neck

Q.2.87 Clinical presentation of malignant nasopharyngeal disease may include

a. lump in the neck
b. abnormal chest X-ray
c. difficulty in swallowing
d. painful neck
e. deafness

Q.2.88 Adenoidectomy is indicated for

a. snoring
b. nasal obstruction
c. secretory otitis media
d. sleep apnoea
e. nasal symptoms with radiological enlarged adenoids

For answers see over

Answers

A.2.85 a. T
           b. T
           c. T
           d. T
           e. T

A.2.86 a. F
           b. T
           c. F
           d. T
           e. F

A.2.87 a. T
           b. F
           c. T
           d. F
           e. T

A.2.88 a. F—Snoring is a symptom of nasal obstruction.
           b. T—When other causes have been excluded.
           c. T
           d. T
           e. T

3. Throat

Q.3.1 Regarding the anatomy and embryology of the oral cavity:

a. It appears about the 10th week in embryonic life
b. Cysts and fistulae are commonly found
c. Sensory innervation of the mobile tongue is by the VIIth nerve
d. The muscles of mastication are supplied by the Vth nerve
e. Lymph drainage to the tongue is bilateral

Q.3.2 Regarding teeth:

a. Adults have 36
b. The third molar and second premolar are missing
c. All permanent teeth have usually erupted by 18 years
d. All deciduous teeth have erupted by 2.5 years
e. Delayed eruption may suggest systemic disease

Q.3.3 Regarding the anatomy of the salivary glands:

a. The glands are mesenchymal in origin
b. The submandibular gland is the first to develop
c. Minor salivary glands are found only in the mouth
d. Saliva can be stimulated by olfactory stimulation.
e. Saliva has a bacteriostatic function

Q.3.4 Regarding the submandibular gland:

a. The lingual nerve runs superior to the duct
b. Damage to the lingual nerve usually recovers
c. The mandibular branch of the facial nerve is in close proximity to the gland
d. The gland is seldom the site of calculi
e. Excision is a simple procedure

For answers see over

Answers

A.3.1 a. T
      b. T
      c. F—Lingual branch of Vth nerve.
      d. T—Mandibular branch of the Vth nerve.
      e. F—Only the tip.

A.3.2 a. F—32 teeth.
      b. T—Children.
      c. F—21 years.
      d. T
      e. T—Such as cretinism.

A.3.3 a. T
      b. F—The parotid at 4–6 weeks, the submandibular gland at 6 +.
      c. F—All over the head and neck area.
      d. T
      e. T

A.3.4 a. F—Below the duct.
      b. F—Seldom recovers.
      c. F—The nerve lies on the outer aspect of the cervical fascia; the gland is deep to the fascia.
      d. F—The most common site of sialolithiasis.
      e. F—Many nerves can be damaged.

Q.3.5   Regarding pharyngeal anatomy:

a. The stapes and part of hyoid are derived from the second pharyngeal pouch
b. The eustachian tube is derived from the second pharyngeal pouch
c. The lower parathyroid gland is derived from the third pharyngeal pouch
d. The pharynx extends from the base of the skull to the level of the 6th cervical vertebra
e. The lower limit of the hypopharynx is the thyroid cartilage

Q.3.6   Regarding the pharynx:

a. Sensation around the tonsil is by the glossopharyngeal nerve
b. Stimulation of the vagus nerve relaxes the cricopharyngeal sphincter
c. The pharyngeal plexus is made up of the vagus and hypoglossal nerves
d. All the muscles of the pharynx are stimulated by the pharyngeal plexus
e. The hypopharynx lies behind the larynx

Q.3.7   Regarding the anatomy of the larynx:

a. The nerves of the IVth and VIth branchial arches innervate the larynx
b. The laryngeal epithelium is ciliated columnar type
c. The superior laryngeal nerve is motor
d. The recurrent laryngeal nerve supplies all the intrinsic muscles of the larynx
e. In men, the larynx lies opposite the 3rd to 6th cervical vertebrae

Q.3.8   Regarding the anatomy of the larynx:

a. The prime function of the larynx is phonation
b. The function of the vocal cords is phonation
c. Aspiration of food is prevented by the epiglottis
d. The right recurrent laryngeal nerve arises in the chest
e. The effects of nerve damage is permanent

For answers see over

Answers

A.3.5 a. T
b. F—The first pouch.
c. T
d. T
e. F—The lower border of the cricoid cartilage.

A.3.6 a. T
b. T
c. F—Glossopharyngeal and vagus nerves.
d. F—All except the stylopharyngeus.
e. F—Only the piriform fossae and the post-cricoid space.

A.3.7 a. T—The superior and recurrent laryngeal nerves.
b. F—The supraglottis is mainly squamous epithelium.
c. F—Mixed nerve-motor to the cricothyroid muscle and sensory to the supraglottis and the piriform fossae.
d. F—All except the cricothyroid muscle.
e. T—Higher in women and children.

A.3.8 a. F—To provide and protect airway functions.
b. T
c. T
d. F
e. F—Compensation results with the passage of time, but the vocal cords may remain permanently paralysed.

Q.3.9   Acute tonsillitis

a. is most commonly caused by β haemolytic streptococcus
b. of non-bacterial origin is often caused by adenoviruses
c. should be treated with erythromycin
d. should be treated with penicillin
e. becomes more frequent with changes of schooling

Q.3.10   Regarding the adenoids:

a. They vary in size from child to child
b. They usually get smaller with age
c. They attain their maximum size by 5 years
d. They usually hypertrophy with tonsillitis
e. The relative size of adenoids to the size of the nasopharynx is most important clinically

Q.3.11   Indications for tonsillectomy include

a. biopsy
b. constant sore throat
c. sleep apnoea
d. recurrent quinsy
e. "tired of antibiotic treatment"

Q.3.12   Regarding chronic pharyngitis in adults:

a. The aetiology is often obscure
b. Blood tests are unhelpful
c. Bacteriology is helpful with management
d. Treatment is best without antibiotics
e. Syphilis may give the same symptoms

Q.3.13   Tonsillectomy may be indicated for

a. "failure to thrive"
b. recurrent septic tonsillitis
c. positive family history
d. quinsy
e. sleep apnoea

For answers see over

Answers

A.3.9   a. T
      b. T
      c. F—Only if allergic to penicillin.
      d. T
      e. T

A.3.10   a. T—Usually from day to day.
       b. T—There is an age resolution pattern.
       c. F—Varies between 3 and 7 years.
       d. T
       e. T

A.3.11   a. T—An absolute indication.
       b. F—Usually fails to cure.
       c. T—When indicated; may be due to massive tonsillar hypertrophy.
       d. T
       e. F—Usually the diagnosis of "tonsillitis" is inaccurate.

A.3.12   a. T
       b. F—Essential to exclude agranulocytosis, leukaemia.
       c. F—Usually sterile.
       d. T
       e. T

A.3.13   a. T
       b. T
       c. F
       d. T
       e. T

Q.3.14 Symptoms of acute tonsillitis

a. include odynophagia (pain on swallowing)
b. include abdominal pains with vomiting
c. include severe earache
d. may herald acute leukaemia
e. indicate a throat swab if diphtheria is suspected

Q.3.15 In the post-tonsillectomy period (at home)

a. antibiotics should be given routinely
b. a jelly and ice cream diet should be given for 2 weeks
c. the patient should remain indoors for 10 days
d. bleeding needs urgent referral to hospital
e. otalgia needs analgesics only

Q.3.16 In infectious mononucleosis (glandular fever)

a. sore throat and lymphadenopathy are the presenting features
b. hepatosplenomegaly is uncommon
c. ampicillin will give a rubelliform rash
d. Guillain-Barré syndrome may develop subsequently
e. diagnosis is by blood tests

Q.3.17 Ulceration of the tonsil

a. can be ignored if asymptomatic
b. is frequently seen in young adults
c. may indicate leukaemia
d. indicates chest X-ray to assist diagnosis
e. always indicates tonsillectomy

Q.3.18 Tumours of the oropharynx may present with the following symptoms:

a. Lymph node in the neck
b. Otalgia
c. Nasal regurgitation of food
d. Dyspnoea
e. Altered (muffled) voice

For answers see over

Answers

A.3.14 a. T
      b. T—Mesenteric adenitis.
      c. T—Referred pain.
      d. T
      e. T

A.3.15 a. F
      b. F—Normal diet as soon as possible.
      c. F—But remain off school/work for approx. two weeks.
      d. T
      e. F—Needs diagnosis first.

A.3.16 a. T
      b. F—Splenomegaly 50%, hepatomegaly 10%.
      c. T—Ampicillin should not be prescribed for sore throats.
      d. T
      e. T—10% will be negative.

A.3.17 a. F—Always investigate.
      b. F
      c. T—A blood test should be done.
      d. T—Lymphoma or myeloma.
      e. T—For histology.

A.3.18 a. T
      b. T
      c. T
      d. T
      e. T

Q.3.19   Histological diagnosis of oropharyngeal tumours includes

a. non-Hodgkin's lymphoma
b. salivary gland tumours
c. squamous cell carcinoma
d. ameloblastoma
e. fibrosarcoma

Q.3.20   Regarding non-Hodgkin's lymphoma of the oropharynx:

a. The tumour is usually part of systemic disease
b. Biopsy can be difficult to interpret
c. An anaplastic result may suggest ectodermal origin
d. Prognosis is poor when associated with adenopathy
e. Surgery is always indicated

Q.3.21   Malignant tumours in the head and neck (children) include

a. lymphoma
b. rhabdomyosarcoma
c. thyroid cancer
d. nasopharyngeal cancer
e. adenocarcinoma of the middle ear

Q.3.22   Retropharyngeal abscess may complicate

a. tonsillitis
b. sinusitis
c. tuberculosis of the cervical vertebrae
d. foreign body perforation of the pharynx
e. chronic otitis media

Q.3.23   In the treatment of sleep related disorders

a. diagnosis by nocturnal polysomnogram
b. medical management is ineffective
c. nasal problems can be ignored
d. tracheostomy may be required
e. snoring may be cured by uvulopharyngopalatoplasty

For answers see over

Answers

A.3.19 a. T—25%.
           b. T—5%.
           c. T—70%.
           d. F
           e. T—But rare.

A.3.20 a. F—Usually localised.
           b. T—May need to be repeated.
           c. T
           d. F
           e. F—Surgical management only required for the diagnosis.

A.3.21 a. T
           b. T—Two age peaks at 2–4 years and 12–15 years.
           c. T
           d. T
           e. F—Very rare even in adults.

A.3.22 a. T
           b. F
           c. T
           d. T
           e. F

A.3.23 a. T
           b. F—Depends on the cause found.
           c. F—May be the cause.
           d. T
           e. T

Q.3.24   Peritonsillar abscess (quinsy)

a. is common in children
b. is synonymous with severe tonsillitis
c. always requires tonsillectomy
d. in adults will produce growth of mixed organisms
e. requires admission to hospital

Q.3.25   Rhabdomyosarcoma

a. presents in the head and neck in more than 50% of patients
b. is a soft tissue sarcoma
c. is usually diagnosed before age 10 years
d. presents as painful masses
e. has a poor prognosis

Q.3.26   Patients with sleep apnoea tend to complain of

a. somnolence during the day
b. overweight
c. interrupted nocturnal sleep
d. intellectual deterioration
e. snoring

Q.3.27   Dental caries

a. is the commonest oral cavity disease
b. risk is increased by high fat diet
c. may be indicated by increased sensitivity to hot and cold fluids
d. of the molars may mimic sinusitis
e. is prevented by fluoride

Q.3.28   Stomatitis

a. is best treated with antibiotics
b. as an acute infection in children is usually due to herpes simplex
c. if recurrent ("cold-sores") is best treated with idoxuridine 1%
d. is not caused by *Candida hyphae*, which is a normal commensal in the mouth
e. treatment with antibiotics is frequently complicated by *Candida*

For answers see over

Answers

A.3.24 a. F—A disease of young adults but may occur in children.
          b. F—Symptoms similar; pathology different.
          c. F—Only if tonsillitis is recurrent.
          d. T
          e. T

A.3.25 a. F—Less than 30%.
          b. T
          c. T—75%.
          d. F—Most commonly painless swelling.
          e. F—Prognosis fair; treatment usually includes chemotherapy and radiotherapy; 5-year survival 50%.

A.3.26 a. T
          b. T—Usually associated.
          c. T
          d. T
          e. T

A.3.27 a. T
          b. F—Carbohydrate diet.
          c. T
          d. T
          e. F—Oral hygiene with removal of plaque.

A.3.28 a. F—Antiseptics.
          b. T
          c. T
          d. T
          e. T

Q.3.29 **Oral lichen planus**

a. is found in more than 10% of the population
b. frequently affects middle aged men
c. is diagnosed with immunological tests
d. appears as symmetrical lesions in the mouth
e. is frequently accompanied by skin lesions

Q.3.30 **Acute erythema multiforme (Stevens Johnson syndrome)**

a. presents as oral ulceration usually accompanied by systemic upsets
b. seldom affects the eyes and skin
c. produces skin lesions characterised by splitting, crusting, erythema and erosions
d. may be precipitated by sulphonamides
e. is diagnosed with immunological tests

Q.3.31 **Oral candidasis**

a. when acute produces white patches that are difficult to remove.
b. may complicate cytotoxic therapy
c. can be confirmed by histology of scrapings
d. is most frequently found in the buccal areas
e. is treated with antifungal creams

Q.3.32 **Regarding premalignant oral cavity lesions:**

a. The white patches are premalignant
b. "Leucoplakia" is not histologically diagnostic of disease
c. Malignant change is inevitable in "leucoplakia"
d. White patches in the floor of mouth need close follow-up
e. Red lesions ("erythroplakia") are safe lesions

Q.3.33 **Temporomandibular joint disorders**

a. often present as pain on opening the mouth
b. are frequently associated with otalgia
c. are commoner in young men
d. can usually be diagnosed on X-ray
e. are usually self limiting

For answers see over

Answers

A.3.29 a. T
        b. F—More commonly affects women.
        c. F—Aetiology unknown.
        d. T
        e. F—Seldom.

A.3.30 a. F—Systemic upset before ulceration.
        b. F
        c. T
        d. T
        e. F—Histology is mainstay of diagnosis—areas of necrosis with eosinophilic colloid changes.

A.3.31 a. F—Only chronic states.
        b. T
        c. T
        d. F—Only the angle of the mouth.
        e. F—Only indicated in symptomatic cases.

A.3.32 a. F—Low risk, but histology always needed.
        b. T—It is purely a clinical descriptive term.
        c. F—Risk 5% over 20 years.
        d. T—Highest risk of tumour transformation.
        e. F—Said to have a higher risk of tumour change.

A.3.33 a. T
        b. T
        c. F—Usually young women
        d. F—Limited help but can exclude organic disease.
        e. T

Q.3.34   Salivary tumours of the mouth

a. present as a non-ulcerative mass.
b. are found frequently in the floor of the mouth
c. are seldom malignant
d. must be treated with excision biopsy
e. are seldom treated with radiotherapy

Q.3.35   Cancer of the lip

a. affects women as frequently as men
b. usually occurs on upper lip
c. is in most cases a basal cell carcinoma
d. is associated with outdoor occupations
e. can in most cases be cured with radiotherapy

Q.3.36   Carcinoma of the oral cavity

a. most frequently involves the buccal area
b. is most commonly an adenocarcinoma
c. is promoted by drinking alcohol and smoking cigarettes
d. is promoted by poor dentition
e. becomes less common with advancing age

Q.3.37   Early symptoms of mouth cancer include

a. difficulty in swallowing with normal barium X-rays
b. pain with "garbled" speech
c. no local symptoms but a lump in the neck
d. earache (in young patients)
e. discomfort on eating spicy food

Q.3.38   Regarding treatment of mouth cancers:

a. Many tumours are advanced on presentation
b. Radiotherapy is the treatment of choice in early disease
c. Chemotherapy is the treatment of choice in early disease
d. Laser therapy may prevent malignant degeneration of leuco-plakia
e. Cryotherapy can help relieve pain

For answers see over

Answers

A.3.34 a. T
   b. F—Hard and soft palate.
   c. F—40%.
   d. T—If possible; sometimes the tumour is too big.
   e. F—Usually combined with surgery.

A.3.35 a. F—The ratio of men to women affected is 8 to 1.
   b. F—Seldom involved.
   c. F—Squamous cell carcinoma.
   d. T
   e. T

A.3.36 a. F—Lateral border of tongue 50%.
   b. F—Squamous carcinoma 75% +.
   c. T
   d. F—No convincing evidence.
   e. F—Advancing age increases risk (at age 74 risk 1 : 1100).

A.3.37 a. T
   b. T
   c. T
   d. F
   e. T—An important symptom in elderly patients.

A.3.38 a. T
   b. T
   c. F—May help shrinkage when used with radiotherapy.
   d. T
   e. T

Q.3.39 Parotitis

a. is the most common infectious disease in childhood
b. is associated with swelling only
c. may cause severe trismus
d. may be managed better with the help of a sialogram
e. causes swelling of the whole gland

Q.3.40 The following drugs can cause enlargement of the parotid gland:

a. Dextropropoxyphene (Distalgesic)
b. High oestrogen contraceptive pill
c. Chlorambucil
d. Vincristine
e. Aldomet

Q.3.41 Treatment of sialectasis may include

a. no treatment
b. marsupialisation of the duct
c. ligation of the duct
d. tympanic neurectomy
e. superficial parotidectomy

Q.3.42 Regarding sialolithasis:

a. The parotid gland is most frequently involved
b. Stones are all radio-opaque
c. Sialogram aids management
d. Removal of the stone leads to cure
e. No treatment may be best treatment

Q.3.43 A discrete lump in the parotid region should always be considered a

a. lymph node
b. parotid cyst
c. parotid neoplasm
d. sarcoidosis
e. inflammatory disease

For answers see over

Answers

A.3.39 a. T—Mumps.
        b. F—Swelling with pain.
        c. T
        d. T
        e. T

A.3.40 a. T
        b. T
        c. F
        d. F
        e. F

A.3.41 a. T—More than 50%.
        b. T—Usually with stone removal.
        c. F
        d. F—Works for about 6 months.
        e. F—Works for about 6 months.

A.3.42 a. F—Usually the submandibular gland (10 : 1).
        b. F—Up to 10% are radiolucent.
        c. F—Only if radiolucent.
        d. F—The cause of development of the stone is a diseased gland
           or a duct stenosis.
        e. T

A.3.43 a. F
        b. F
        c. T
        d. F
        e. F

Q.3.44 **Sjögren's syndrome symptoms include**

a. dry mouth (xerostomia)
b. dry eyes (xerophthalmia)
c. parotitis
d. joint pains
e. rheumatoid arthritis

Q.3.45 **Sjögren's syndrome**

a. is diagnosed with blood tests
b. can be treated symptomatically with steroids
c. is associated with increased risk of lymphoma
d. is associated with raised prevalence of HLA A1 and HLA B8
e. is associated with absence of filamentary keratitis

Q.3.46 **Salivary neoplasms**

a. have an incidence of 20 per million per year in the UK
b. present in the submandibular gland in 60% of cases
c. of the parotid gland are benign in 80% of cases
d. are never found in the middle ear
e. should preferably be treated with radiotherapy

Q.3.47 **The following clinical signs suggest that a parotid lump is malignant:**

a. Discrete mass in the cheek
b. Multinodularity
c. Ulceration of the skin
d. Distortion of the parapharyngeal space
e. Facial nerve palsy or division palsy

Q.3.48 **Regarding salivary gland tumours—parotid:**

a. Clinically benign lumps are always benign
b. Mobile lumps are always lateral to the facial nerve
c. Facial nerve paralysis always confirms malignancy
d. Lumpectomy is the best treatment
e. Recurrences even in benign disease may appear after an interval of up to 15 years.

For answers see over

Answers

A.3.44 a. T
          b. T
          c. F
          d. F—Polymyositis.
          e. T

A.3.45 a. F—Labial biopsy necessary.
          b. F
          c. T—1:5 risk.
          d. T—But not a diagnostic test.
          e. F—Keratoconjunctivitis is a feature of the disease.

A.3.46 a. T
          b. F—80% are found in the parotid gland.
          c. T
          d. F
          e. F

A.3.47 a. T—Location is helpful: lesions in the cheek are more likely to be malignant than benign.
          b. T
          c. T
          d. F—Lesions usually benign; however, should be excised as "malignant".
          e. T

A.3.48 a. F—Up to 25% turn out malignant.
          b. F—Up to 15% are in close proximity to the nerve.
          c. F—Suggests malignant; tissue diagnosis necessary.
          d. F—Higher risk of nerve damage and recurrence.
          e. T

Q.3.49 Pleomorphic adenoma of the parotid

a. is the commonest of all benign tumours
b. can be diagnosed clinically with certainty
c. is always surrounded by a complete capsule
d. should be excised with a wide margin
e. when recurrent can easily be treated by further surgery

Q.3.50 Warthin's tumour of the parotid

a. is seldom bilateral
b. is primarily a tumour of men
c. is usually located in the tail of the parotid
d. usually makes up 10% of benign parotid tumours
e. seldom recurs after surgery

Q.3.51 Recurrent pleomorphic adenoma

a. is usually due to inadequate surgery
b. usually results from tumour rupture at the time of excision
c. tends to occur in younger patients
d. is less likely if tumour is removed by superficial parotidectomy.
e. can be prevented by radiotherapy following incomplete surgery

Q.3.52 Useful investigations of suspected salivary neoplasms include

a. clinical examination
b. sialogram
c. computed tomographic scan
d. fine needle aspiration
e. incisional biopsy

Q.3.53 Late complications of parotid surgery include

a. salivary fistula
b. gustatory hyperhydrosis (Frey's syndrome)
c. anaesthesia of the pinna
d. greater auricular neuroma
e. recurrence of the tumour

For answers see over

Answers

A.3.49 a. T
　　　　b. F—Suspected only.
　　　　c. F—Pseudocapsule.
　　　　d. T
　　　　e. F—Very difficult; may even have become malignant.

A.3.50 a. F—10% bilateral.
　　　　b. T
　　　　c. T
　　　　d. T
　　　　e. T

A.3.51 a. T
　　　　b. T
　　　　c. T
　　　　d. T
　　　　e. F—Should be reserved for recurrences.

A.3.52 a. T
　　　　b. F—usually adds no additional information to clinical diagnosis
　　　　　 and is a painful procedure.
　　　　c. T
　　　　d. T—But only if diagnostic.
　　　　e. F—To be condemned.

A.3.53 a. T
　　　　b. T
　　　　c. T
　　　　d. T
　　　　e. T

Q.3.54 Malignant salivary gland tumours

a. are more commonly found in the minor salivary glands
b. are usually located in the oral cavity
c. have a peak incidence in 7th decade in men.
d. in children are more commonly mucoepidermoid cancer
e. have an incidence of 3–4 per million

Q.3.55 In the management of malignant salivary gland tumours

a. open biopsy will aid diagnosis
b. computed tomographic scanning will help delineate the extent of the disease
c. the facial nerve can usually be spared
d. radical excision is the treatment of choice
e. postoperative radiotherapy may reduce risk of local recurrences

Q.3.56 Prognosis of salivary malignancy

a. depends on the histological type
b. depends on the site of the lesion
c. is best when malignant change is seen in a previously benign lesion
d. is good for acinic-cell carcinoma
e. is poor in adenoid cystic carcinoma; recurrences herald a rapid death.

Q.3.57 Regarding midline neck swellings:

a. They are most frequently thyroid
b. All thyroglossal duct cysts should be excised
c. Submental dermoids must be differentiated from thyroglossal cysts
d. 20% of submental lumps are deep to the mylohyoid
e. Thyroid isotope scan is the investigation of choice

For answers see over

Answers

A.3.54 a. T
          b. T
          c. F—7th decade in women.
          d. T
          e. T

A.3.55 a. F—To be condemned.
          b. T
          c. F
          d. T
          e. T

A.3.56 a. T
          b. T
          c. F—Usually very bad.
          d. T
          e. F—Can usually live for many years with recurrent disease.

A.3.57 a. T
          b. T
          c. F—Management is excision.
          d. T
          e. F—Ultrasound scan.

Q.3.58 **Regarding neck lumps in children:**

a. Cervical adenitis is usually bacterial
b. A persistent lump may be lymphoma
c. Antibiotics help to resolve the lump
d. If associated with functional interference urgent referral is required
e. If located at the thyroid level may be malignant

Q.3.59 **Thyroglossal duct cysts**

a. occur mostly in adults
b. present as a lump at the hyoid level
c. move on swallowing because they are attached to the tongue
d. are cured by excision
e. may be located in the posterior tongue

Q.3.60 **Regarding branchial cysts:**

a. Peak incidence is in young adults
b. Men are more commonly affected than women
c. Intermittent swelling is frequently found
d. They are located at the upper third of the sternomastoid muscle
e. Excision may reveal a sinus tract to the tonsil

Q.3.61 **Regarding thyroid neoplasms:**

a. They may be familial
b. Follicular carcinoma is the most common type
c. Age of presentation is an important prognostic factor
d. Nodal involvement in papillary carcinoma reduces survival
e. A non-functioning thyroid nodule should be excised

For answers see over

Answers

A.3.58 a. F—Viral.
 b. T
 c. F
 d. T
 e. T

A.3.59 a. F—More than 50% present before 2 years of age.
 b. T
 c. F—Because they are attached to the hyoid bone.
 d. F—Recurrences frequent if the body of the hyoid not removed (Sistrunk's operation).
 e. T—Need to consider lingual thyroid.

A.3.60 a. F—The third decade.
 b. T—60%.
 c. T
 d. T
 e. F—Very rarely found.

A.3.61 a. T—Autosomal dominant medullary carcinoma.
 b. F—60% papillary.
 c. T
 d. F
 e. T

Q.3.62 Thyroid surgery

a. may result in stridor
b. may cause temporary hypocalcaemia
c. should be followed up for life
d. may damage the superior laryngeal nerve without causing symptoms
e. may be complicated by damage to the recurrent laryngeal nerve, which usually recovers by 6 months

Q.3.63 Regarding neck lumps:

a. Primary tumours need to be sought before biopsy
b. Squamous carcinoma is frequently found
c. Incision biopsy is adequate management
d. Malignant lumps are best treated with radiotherapy
e. Neck dissection is seldom indicated

Q.3.64 Dysphagia means

a. difficulty with swallowing
b. a sensation of discomfort in the throat
c. discomfort initiated by pharyngeal movement
d. discomfort relieved by swallowing
e. discomfort related to swallowing

Q.3.65 Globus pharyngeus is characterised by

a. difficulty in swallowing
b. a sensation of a lump in the throat
c. tightness of the chest
d. anxiety
e. hyperventilation

Q.3.66 Important symptoms suggestive of oesophageal disease include

a. sensation of a lump in the throat on swallowing saliva
b. difficulty in swallowing
c. food regurgitation
d. pain on swallowing
e. paroxysmal coughing and spluttering

For answers see over

Answers

A.3.62 a. T—Bilateral recurrent laryngeal palsy.
        b. T
        c. T
        d. F—Limits the singing voice.
        e. T—If recovery is going to occur.

A.3.63 a. T
        b. T
        c. F—To be condemned.
        d. F—Excision.
        e. F—Indicated for metastatic head and neck squamous cell carcinoma.

A.3.64 a. T
        b. F
        c. T
        d. F
        e. T

A.3.65 a. F
        b. T
        c. T
        d. T
        e. T

A.3.66 a. F—Usually occurs in pharyngeal disease.
        b. T
        c. T
        d. F—Odynophagia is a symptom of pharyngeal disease.
        e. F—Overspilling into the larynx. The cause must be diagnosed.

Q.3.67 **Investigation of swallowing disorders must include**

a. history of symptoms
b. observation of swallow
c. cineradiology of swallow
d. indirect laryngoscopy
e. oesophagoscopy

Q.3.68 **Foreign body ingested in the upper digestive tract may be impacted or located in the**

a. tonsil
b. valleculae
c. cricopharyngeal area
d. level of the aortic arch
e. stomach

Q.3.69 **Oesophageal foreign bodies**

a. need to be removed in most cases
b. are usually held up at the cricopharyngeus
c. cause choking, excessive salivation and dysphagia
d. seldom cause perforation
e. if radio-opaque need contrast to locate level

Q.3.70 **Congenital oesophageal atresia**

a. is an uncommon congenital disorder
b. is associated with other abnormalities
c. is suggested if polyhydramnios is present
d. will not allow the passage of a catheter below 15 cm
e. requires early surgical correction

For answers see over

Answers

A.3.67 a. T
      b. T
      c. T
      d. T
      e. T—Usually by now you should have a diagnosis.

A.3.68 a. T
      b. T
      c. T
      d. T
      e. F—Gastro-oesophageal junction.

A.3.69 a. F—Over 90% pass eventually.
      b. T—80%.
      c. T
      d. F
      e. F—Need anterio-posterior and lateral films.

A.3.70 a. F—1:4000 live births.
      b. T—40%.
      c. T—30%.
      d. F—More usually 10 cm.
      e. T

Q.3.71 **Gastro-oesophageal reflux (in children)**

    a. is commonly found in the newborn

    b. is associated with a sliding hernia

    c. may be accompanied by complications if projectile vomiting present

    d. may be associated with recurrent respiratory tract infections in older children

    e. does not usually require endoscopy.

Q.3.72 **A carcinoma of the gastro-oesophageal junction**

    a. may arise as a complication of achalasia of the cardia

    b. may mimic achalasia of the cardia on barium swallow

    c. may present as dysphagia at the cricoid level

    d. may be an incidental finding in bolus obstruction

    e. can be confidently differentiated from a benign stricture on barium X-ray

Q.3.73 **Tumours of the hypopharynx are virtually all**

    a. benign

    b. squamous cell carcinoma

    c. associated with cervical adenopathy

    d. in young patients

    e. unsuitable for curative treatment

Q.3.74 **The aetiology of postcricoid carcinoma is associated with**

    a. sideropenic anaemia

    b. smoking

    c. alcohol

    d. previous radiotherapy in the neck

    e. reflux oesophagitis

For answers see over

Answers

A.3.71 a. T
            b. T
            c. F—? Pyloric stenosis.
            d. T
            e. F—Should always be performed.

A.3.72 a. T
            b. T
            c. T
            d. T
            e. F

A.3.73 a. F
            b. T—95% of all tumours.
            c. T
            d. F—Usually middle aged.
            e. T

A.3.74 a. T—Up to 50%.
            b. F
            c. F
            d. T
            e. F

Q.3.75 Symptoms suggestive of hypopharyngeal disease may include

a. "something in the throat"
b. lump in the neck
c. nasal regurgitation of food
d. dysphagia
e. "sore throat"

Q.3.76 Prognosis of hypopharyngeal cancer depends on

a. age of patient
b. presence of metastases
c. length of tumour
d. previous sideropenic anaemia
e. invasion of the larynx

Q.3.77 Regarding hypopharyngeal cancers:

a. Overall survival is poor
b. The aim of treatment is rapid relief of symptoms
c. Radiotherapy is the treatment of choice
d. Surgery is associated with high mortality
e. Symptoms are not best relieved with radiotherapy

Q.3.78 Symptoms of a pharyngeal pouch include

a. dysphagia
b. dysphonia
c. odynophagia
d. paroxysmal coughing
e. foul taste in the mouth

Q.3.79 Pharyngeal pouch

a. is diagnosed with radiology
b. is usually suggested by symptoms
c. may be a coincidental finding on X-ray
d. always needs treatment
e. is associated with cancer

For answers see over

Answers

A.3.75 a. T
            b. T
            c. F
            d. T
            e. T

A.3.76 a. T
            b. T
            c. T
            d. F
            e. T

A.3.77 a. T—2 year survival 15%.
            b. T
            c. F—Tends to exacerbate the local symptoms.
            d. F
            e. T

A.3.78 a. T
            b. F—Hoarseness.
            c. F
            d. T
            e. T

A.3.79 a. T
            b. T
            c. T
            d. F
            e. F—However, cancer needs to be out ruled by endoscopy.

Q.3.80 **Regarding paediatric airway problems:**
a. Stridor is a diagnosis
b. Wheeze is noisy inspiratory breathing
c. Stertor is partial airway obstruction above the level of the larynx
d. Croup means noisy breathing
e. Mixed noisy breathing means a lesion located at the level of the larynx

Q.3.81 **Regarding congenital laryngeal disease:**
a. The incidence is unknown
b. Congenital stridor always suggests a laryngeal cause
c. More than one congenital abnormality is often found
d. Symptoms may be part of extended syndrome
e. Endoscopy should always be done to establish diagnosis

Q.3.82 **Abnormal cry in childhood may suggest**
a. laryngomalacia
b. laryngeal cysts
c. laryngeal webs
d. vocal cord paralysis
e. subglottic stenosis

Q.3.83 **Feeding problems may be encountered in the following paediatric laryngeal disorders:**
a. Laryngomalacia
b. Laryngeal cyst
c. Vocal cord palsy
d. Laryngotracheal clefts
e. Laryngeal web

For answers see over

Answers

A.3.80   a. F—It is a symptom meaning noisy breathing.
           b. F—It is a noise located at the level of alveoli or bronchi.
           c. T
           d. T
           e. T

A.3.81   a. T—Estimated 1:10 000 to 1:50 000 births.
           b. F—60% only; other lesions may be located in the trachea and bronchi.
           c. T—Up to 40% have more congenital lesions.
           d. T
           e. T

A.3.82   a. F
           b. T—Occasionally.
           c. T
           d. T
           e. F

A.3.83   a. F
           b. F
           c. T—In the early stages only.
           d. T
           e. F

Q.3.84 In recent-onset acute laryngeal airway problems in previously normal children the differential diagnosis includes
a. trauma
b. glandular fever
c. foreign body
d. retropharyngeal abscess
e. diphtheria

Q.3.85 Retropharyngeal abscess (in children)
a. presents as airway obstruction
b. needs to be differentiated from foreign body
c. is frequently seen in older children
d. is best diagnosed on clinical history and examination
e. is managed by early use of antibiotics

Q.3.86 Management of childhood airway obstructive problems
a. requires correct diagnosis
b. is a simple clinical problem
c. requires a thorough family history
d. requires the securing of a safe airway
e. may require a tracheostomy

Q.3.87 Regarding antibiotics in paediatric airway problems:
a. Ampicillin is indicated for epiglottitis
b. There is seldom a need in laryngotracheobronchitis
c. Secondary bacterial infection is best treated with flucloxacillin
d. Foreign body should first be excluded
e. Oral preparations are acceptable to the parents

Q.3.88 Laryngotracheobronchitis
a. most frequently affects 4–5-year-olds
b. causes children to be restless and pink
c. may not affect the voice
d. is caused by parainfluenza virus type I
e. is frequently confused with epiglottitis

For answers see over

Answers

A.3.84 a. T
b. T
c. T
d. T
e. T

A.3.85 a. T
b. T
c. F—Usually under 4 years.
d. F—Lateral soft tissue of the neck X-ray is important; may sometimes need examination under a general anaesthetic.
e. F—Surgical decompression should be carried out first, but antibiotics are also required.

A.3.86 a. T
b. F—May result in death if mismanaged.
c. F—Usually a waste of time.
d. T
e. T

A.3.87 a. T—Chloramphenicol may be required if the organism is resistant to ampicillin.
b. T—Humidification usually works rapidly if diagnosis is correct.
c. T
d. T
e. F—Treatment is for the patient not the parents; parenteral treatment is rapid and preferable.

A.3.88 a. F—18 months.
b. T—Epiglottitis patients are pale and quiet and look terrified.
c. F—Always affected.
d. T
e. F—40 times more frequent.

Q.3.89 Laryngomalacia

a. means tightening of the laryngeal tissues
b. is located throughout the larynx
c. is uncommon in females
d. accounts for more than 70% of chronic laryngeal airway problems
e. usually resolves after age 12 months

Q.3.90 Subglottic stenosis

a. lies at the level of the vocal cords
b. may be congenital
c. causes inspiratory stridor
d. is diagnosed mainly by endoscopy
e. if severe requires surgery

Q.3.91 Acute Epiglottitis

a. seldom results in death
b. is most commonly caused by *Haemophilus influenzae* type B
c. frequently presents in the autumn months
d. most commonly occurs between ages 5 and 6 years
e. may be preceded by an upper respiratory tract infection

Q.3.92 Foreign body inhalations

a. are associated with a history of choking followed by paroxysmal coughing
b. occur before age 3 years in 75% of cases
c. may cause "sudden deaths" of infancy
d. can be excluded if a wheeze is present
e. are suggested by coughing, wheeze and choking

For answers see over

Answers

A.3.89 a. F—The term means a floppy larynx.
          b. F—Flaccidity of the supraglottis is the main pathology.
          c. F—Equal sex distribution.
          d. T
          e. T—Maximal symptoms at 9–12 months.

A.3.90 a. F—At the level of the cricoid cartilage.
          b. T
          c. T—In extensive lesions may be biphasic.
          d. T
          e. T—Laser therapy or tracheostomy with laryngotracheoplasty.

A.3.91 a. F—3%–4% mortality.
          b. T
          c. F—Winter months.
          d. F—3–4 years.
          e. T—Up to 33%.

A.3.92 a. T
          b. T
          c. T
          d. F—Foreign body needs to be excluded.
          e. T

Q.3.93 **Regarding investigation of suspected inhaled foreign body:**
a. Clinical examination is seldom helpful
b. Obstructive emphysema on chest X-ray suggests a foreign body
c. The majority come to rest in the left main bronchus
d. Foreign bodies are always seen on chest X-ray
e. Endoscopy is indicated if other tests are unhelpful

Q.3.94 **Juvenile laryngeal papillomatosis**
a. is found only in the larynx
b. usually presents before age 4 years
c. presents as hoarseness or abnormal cry
d. occurs in children born by caesarean section
e. can be cured with surgery

Q.3.95 **Paediatric tracheostomy**
a. is most frequently indicated for congenital laryngeal abnormalities
b. should be considered when intubation is protracted
c. is indicated before age 1 year in more than 50% of cases
d. can easily be performed in the intensive care unit
e. requires a "window" to aid changing of the tubes

Q.3.96 **Regarding tracheostomy in children:**
a. The procedure is best reserved for difficult cases
b. Patients can be nursed safely in the open ward
c. Complications can include a pneumothorax
d. Dislodgement of the tube may easily occur
e. The procedure is best performed by a paediatric laryngologist

Q.3.97 **Regarding complications of tracheostomy:**
a. Surgical emphysema is uncommon
b. Accidental decannulation may be fatal
c. Chest infections are prevented by tracheostomy
d. The risk can be reduced by frequent tube changes
e. Peristomal bleeding should always be considered serious

For answers see over

Answers

A.3.93 a. F—If there is clinical suspicion examination is often positive.
        b. T
        c. F—Usually the right.
        d. F
        e. T

A.3.94 a. F—Have been detected in the oesophagus and trachea.
        b. T
        c. T
        d. F—Only vaginal delivery.
        e. F—Surgery is a treatment but may not be curative; repeated removal is usually necessary.

A.3.95 a. T
        b. T
        c. T
        d. F—Should be performed in the operating theatre.
        e. F—This may predispose to tracheal stenosis.

A.3.96 a. F—Depends on local expertise.
        b. F—Initially need experienced and individual nursing.
        c. T
        d. T
        e. T

A.3.97 a. F—Need to check the position of the tube.
        b. T
        c. F—Frequent complication.
        d. F—The risk is increased during the early phase before a definite track is established.
        e. T

Q.3.98 Decannulation of the tracheostomised child

a. is always possible
b. requires consideration of endoscopy at 6-month intervals
c. may require radiology if difficulty arises
d. should always be carried out in hospital
e. requires surgical closure

Q.3.99 Cystic fibrosis

a. affects 1:20 000 births in the UK
b. symptoms are due to hormonal imbalance
c. may present with staphylococcal pneumonia
d. should be suspected in an infant with nasal polyps and sinusitis
e. diagnosed in one child indicates need for screening of siblings

Q.3.100 Symptoms of laryngeal dysfunction include

a. loss of voice
b. difficulty in swallowing
c. sensation of something in the throat
d. increasing difficulty with breathing
e. choking on food

Q.3.101 Investigation of a laryngeal disorder is best assessed by

a. computed tomographic scanning
b. chest X-ray
c. thyroid function studies
d. indirect laryngoscopy
e. laryngostroboscopy

Q.3.102 Radiology of the larynx is

a. better than clinical examination
b. always diagnostic
c. sometimes useful in identification of foreign body
d. helpful in cancer diagnosis
e. best performed by magnetic resonance imaging

For answers see over

Answers

A.3.98 a. F—Depends on the indication for tracheostomy.
      b. T
      c. T—May demonstrate substomal stenosis or granuloma.
      d. T
      e. F—Uncommon in early cases. However, if the tracheostomy
         has been present for more than 3 months surgical closure may
         be indicated.

A.3.99 a. F—1 : 2000 births.
      b. F—Abnormality of the exocrine glandular secretions.
      c. T
      d. T
      e. T

A.3.100 a. T
       b. F
       c. T
       d. T
       e. F

A.3.101 a. F
       b. F
       c. F
       d. T
       e. T—If available.

A.3.102 a. F
       b. F
       c. T
       d. F
       e. F—Currently computed tomographic scans

Q.3.103 **Radiology of the larynx may include**

a. xerograms
b. computed tomographic scanning
c. ultrasound
d. isotope scanning
e. magnetic resonance imaging

Q.3.104 **Ossification of the laryngeal cartilages**

a. seldom occurs before the third decade
b. is frequently confused with a foreign body
c. usually starts in the cricoid cartilage
d. seldom occurs in the thyrohyoid ligament
e. is frequently found in the epiglottis

Q.3.105 **Radiological thickening of the prevertebral soft tissue may be**

a. normal in children
b. suggestive of retropharyngeal abscess
c. due to rotation of the patient
d. suggestive of a postcricoid carcinoma in an adult with symptoms
e. ignored

Q.3.106 **Computed tomography of the larynx**

a. is better than clinical examination
b. can diagnose early cancer
c. is helpful in the management of laryngeal trauma
d. can help in the diagnosis of laryngeal palsy
e. can identify the pre-epiglottic space

Q.3.107 **Voice assessment may include**

a. phonetograph
b. stroboscopy
c. laryngograph
d. psychological profile
e. auscultation

For answers see over

Answers

A.3.103 a. T
           b. T
           c. F
           d. F
           e. T

A.3.104 a. T
           b. T
           c. F—Thyroid cartilage.
           d. F—Frequently found.
           e. F

A.3.105 a. T
           b. T
           c. T
           d. T
           e. F—May need further investigation depending on the symptoms and the age of the patient.

A.3.106 a. F
           b. F
           c. T
           d. F
           e. T

A.3.107 a. T
           b. T
           c. T
           d. T
           e. T—Listening to the voice.

Q.3.108   **Disorders of voice are in many cases**

a. intermittent
b. psychogenic in origin
c. reversed if the patient understands the cause
d. due to thyroid disorders
e. organic in children

Q.3.109   **Acute laryngitis**

a. is usually viral in origin
b. is associated with discomfort in the throat
c. usually lasts for 3 weeks
d. requires local treatment only
e. requires antibiotic treatment if local symptoms are protracted

Q.3.110   **Voice production (phonation) requires**

a. the lower respiratory system
b. the larynx
c. a resonator system
d. a central nervous system
e. the thyroid gland

Q.3.111   **Specific infectious causes of hoarseness include**

a. tuberculosis
b. candida
c. Wegener's granulomatosis
d. sarcoidosis
e. syphilis

Q.3.112   **Chronic hoarseness**

a. is always infectious in origin
b. lasting more than 6 months is serious
c. may be an early sign of malignancy
d. can be caused by thyroid disease
e. requires inspection of the vocal cords

For answers see over

Answers

A.3.108 a. T
            b. T
            c. T
            d. F
            e. F—Usually functional.

A.3.109 a. T
            b. T
            c. F—Less than a week.
            d. T—Analgesics.
            e. F—Usually do not speed up recovery.

A.3.110 a. T—Good lungs.
            b. T
            c. F—Only help to modulate the voice.
            d. T
            e. F

A.3.111 a. T
            b. T
            c. F
            d. F
            e. T

A.3.112 a. F
            b. F—If more than 4 weeks may be due to cancer.
            c. T
            d. T—However, inspection of the vocal cords is necessary if hoarseness persists.
            e. T

Q.3.113 **Regarding chronic laryngitis:**

    a. The dominant symptom is discomfort of the throat

    b. Middle-aged men are the most commonly affected

    c. Chronic non-specific inflammation is found

    d. Symptoms tend to relapse

    e. Long-term follow-up is indicated

Q.3.114 **"Laryngitis" following laryngeal intubation (hoarseness)**

    a. is usually complained of immediately

    b. is seldom serious

    c. affects women more frequently than men

    d. can often be cured by means of reassurance

    e. requires referral for laryngoscopy

Q.3.115 **Oedema of the vocal cords (Reinke's oedema)**

    a. is a benign soft tissue tumour

    b. affects women more frequently than men

    c. is in many cases associated with smoking

    d. can be helped with speech therapy, which eases hoarseness

    e. always indicates surgical excision

Q.3.116 **Acute laryngeal trauma**

    a. is most frequently associated with blunt injuries of the neck

    b. usually affects teenage girls

    c. is seldom associated with other injuries

    d. requires airway management as the initial priority

    e. requires a chest X-ray if surgical emphysema in the neck tissues

Q.3.117 **Laryngeal stenosis**

    a. is usually due to prolonged intubation

    b. is subglottic if due to systemic disease

    c. may be caused by a high tracheostomy

    d. if subglottic can be successfully treated

    e. does not preclude the achieving of a good voice (by surgical means)

For answers see over

Answers

A.3.113 a. F—Hoarseness.
  b. T
  c. T
  d. T
  e. T—There is a risk of change to malignancy.

A.3.114 a. F—May take months.
  b. F—May be a malignancy missed at the time of intubation.
  c. T
  d. F—Only if there is no cause found at laryngoscopy.
  e. T—To make a diagnosis.

A.3.115 a. F—Congestion of the mucosa of the cord.
  b. T
  c. T
  d. T
  e. F—Only if the voice does not respond to speech therapy.

A.3.116 a. T
  b. F—Young men.
  c. F—Major other injury is to the cervical vertebrae.
  d. T
  e. F—Only as part of the assessment rather than as a diagnostic test.

A.3.117 a. T
  b. F—Usually glottic/supraglottic.
  c. T
  d. F
  e. T

Q.3.118 **Regarding paralysis of the recurrent laryngeal nerve:**

a. There is a high risk that the cause is a malignancy
b. In many patients no cause can be found
c. A chest X-ray can determine the diagnosis
d. Speech therapy is not usually indicated
e. Surgery can speed up recovery of voice

Q.3.119 **Bilateral abductor palsy of the vocal cords is uncommon but may be caused by**

a. thyrotoxicosis
b. thyroidectomy
c. myasthenia gravis
d. carcinoma of the cervical oesophagus
e. carcinoma of the thyroid

Q.3.120 **In surgical rehabilitation of vocal cord palsy**

a. the paralysed vocal cord can be augmented by injection of Teflon paste
b. aspiration is a contraindication
c. voice improvement is "normal"
d. voice improvement is rapid and permanent
e. age and aetiology modify management

Q.3.121 **Granulomata of the larynx**

a. are usually due to trauma
b. requires histological diagnosis
c. has hoarseness as a late symptom
d. can be cured by surgical excision
e. may be caused by reflux

Q.3.122 **Tracheostomy in adults**

a. is usually to aid ventilation
b. may result in cardiac arrest
c. is indicated in bilateral vocal cord palsy
d. can seldom be done under local anaesthetic
e. is seldom obstructed by the thyroid isthmus

For answers see over

Answers

A.3.118 a. T—Up to 30% in left cord palsy.
b. T—10% or more.
c. F—The diagnosis can only be made by viewing the vocal cord movement.
d. F—May speed up compensatory vocal cord movement.
e. T—But usually wait for 6 months for spontaneous vocal cord compensation. Augmentation of the cord usually by injection of Teflon.

A.3.119 a. F
b. T
c. F
d. T
e. T

A.3.120 a. T
b. F
c. F
d. T
e. T

A.3.121 a. T—Intubation.
b. T
c. F—In the majority hoarseness is the only symptom.
d. F—Depends on the aetiology.
e. T

A.3.122 a. T
b. T
c. T
d. F—The majority can safely be carried out under local anaesthetic.
e. F—Needs to be divided in all cases.

Q.3.123 Regarding tumours of the larynx:

a. Benign tumours are common
b. Malignant tumours are rare
c. Symptoms may differentiate benign from malignant
d. Chondromata of the larynx are diagnosed by indirect laryngoscopy
e. All malignant tumours present as non-ulcerative lesions

Q.3.124 Cancer of the larynx

a. is most frequently an adenocarcinoma
b. makes up approximately 1% of all malignancy in the UK
c. has an overall cure rate of over 50%
d. affects women more frequently than men
e. becomes more common with increasing age

Q.3.125 Regarding symptoms of laryngeal disease:

a. Intermittent hoarseness can be ignored
b. Cancer needs to be excluded in chronic hoarseness
c. Increasing dyspnoea suggests a supraglottic cancer
d. Pain is a common symptom of cancer
e. Halitosis may be a presenting symptom of cancer

Q.3.126 Regarding squamous carcinoma of the larynx:

a. Most carcinomas are located in the supraglottis
b. Cervical lymphadenopathy is common with glottic cancers
c. The presence of cervical lymphadenopathy is a major prognostic factor
d. Biopsy is essential for management
e. Radiotherapy is the most frequent treatment used

Q.3.127 Management of laryngeal cancer frequently includes

a. chemotherapy
b. surgery
c. radiotherapy
d. cryotherapy
e. no treatment

For answers see over

Answers

A.3.123   a. F
  b. F—90% of all laryngeal tumours are malignant.
  c. F—Hoarseness is the most common symptom whether due to a benign or a malignant lesion.
  d. F—Usually need radiology.
  e. F—Sarcomas and lymphomas.

A.3.124   a. F—Squamous cell carcinoma (85%).
  b. T—Approximately 1600 new cases per year.
  c. T
  d. F—10 times more men than women are affected.
  e. T

A.3.125   a. F
  b. F
  c. T—May also be the site of a glottic/subglottic/tracheal lesion.
  d. F
  e. T—Especially in supraglottic lesions.

A.3.126   a. F—Glottis (60%).
  b. F
  c. T
  d. T—Not the neck, the primary larynx!
  e. T

A.3.127   a. F
  b. T
  c. T
  d. F
  e. F—The majority are fit for treatment.

Q.3.128 **Radiotherapy for carcinoma of the larynx**

a. preserves voice function
b. is indicated when pain is severe
c. can be repeated for recurrences
d. is indicated for early tumours
e. can be considered when patients refuse surgery

Q.3.129 **Reactions following laryngeal radiotherapy**

a. are usually due to severe mucositis
b. can be minimised by stopping smoking and alcohol drinking
c. can be helped by analgesics
d. include troublesome nausea
e. include laryngeal stenosis as a late complication

Q.3.130 **Indications for laryngeal surgery include**

a. early tumours of the larynx
b. persistent aspiration following radiotherapy
c. chondrosarcoma of the thyroid cartilage
d. recurrent tumours following radiotherapy
e. non-Hodgkin's lymphoma of the larynx

Q.3.131 **Complications following total laryngectomy may include**

a. hypercalcaemia
b. reflux oesophagitis
c. hypothyroidism
d. anosmia
e. aspiration of food

Q.3.132 **Management of vocal cord nodules should include**

a. advising the patient to stop talking
b. advising speech therapy
c. advising the patient to whisper only
d. immediate admission for surgery
e. antibiotics

For answers see over

Answers

A.3.128 a. T
      b. F—Usually suggests cartilage involvement.
      c. F
      d. T
      e. T—But may not be complementary to surgery.

A.3.129 a. T
      b. T—During treatment only.
      c. T
      d. F—Seldom a problem.
      e. T

A.3.130 a. F
      b. T
      c. T
      d. T
      e. F—Local radiotherapy with or without chemotherapy.

A.3.131 a. F
      b. F
      c. T
      d. T
      e. F

A.3.132 a. F—Not any use on its own.
      b. T
      c. F
      d. F—Recurrences frequent.
      e. F

Q.3.133 **Functional voice disorders exist when**

a. all the laryngeal functions of the larynx are abnormal
b. no abnormality can be demonstrated to account for the voice disorder
c. the voice is abnormal but cough is normal
d. cough is abnormal but the voice is normal
e. swallowing is abnormal but the voice and cough are normal

For answers see over

Answers

A.3.133 a. F
        b. T
        c. T—But needs laryngoscopic examination.
        d. F
        e. F